To my amazing children,

Teaching you to be healthy, active and happy is the greatest gift I can give.

Having you learn this by following my lead will be my greatest accomplishment.

SIMPLE MEALS

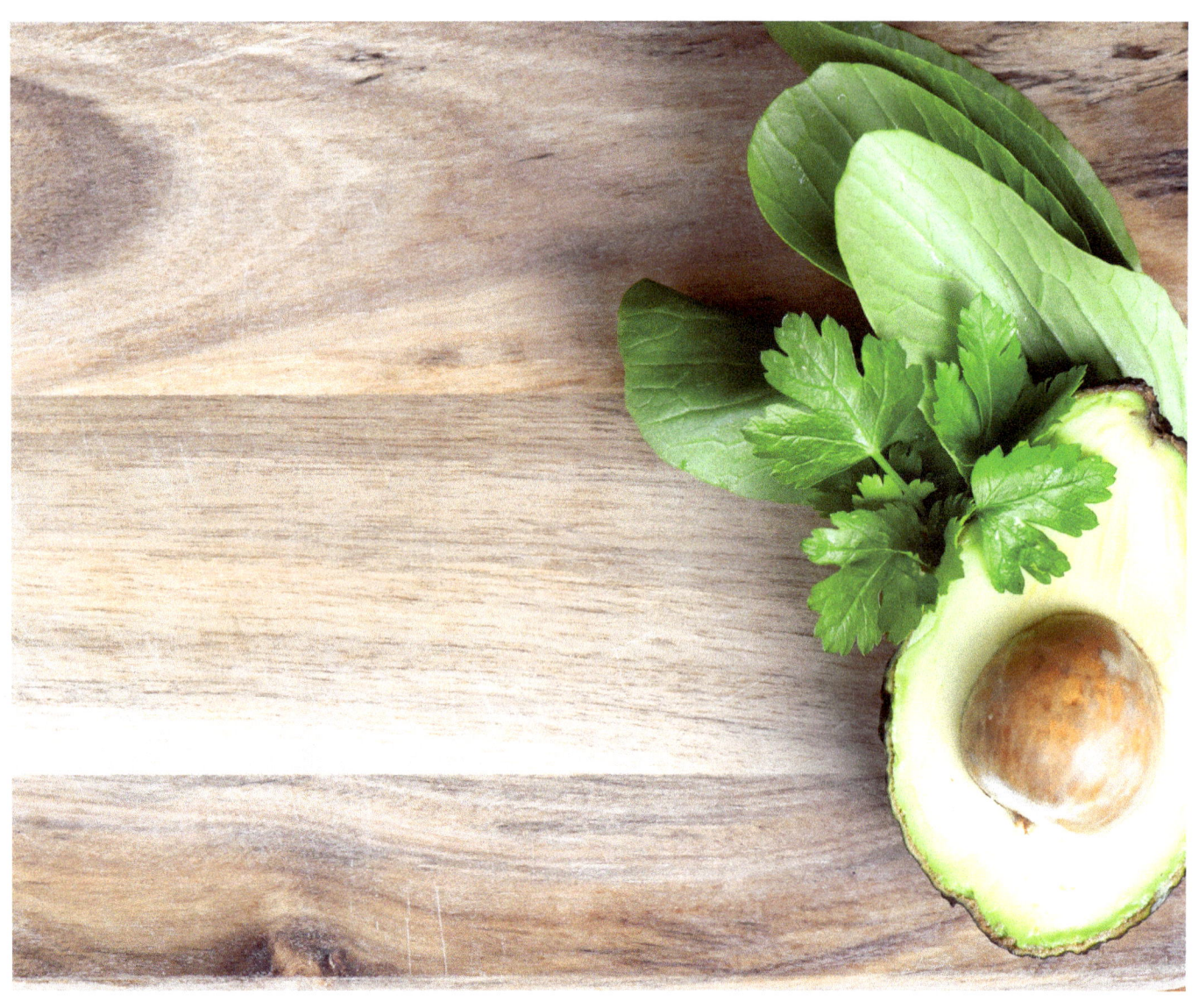

Nut and Oat Crunch

You'll love this cereal so much that you would want it everyday for breakfast.

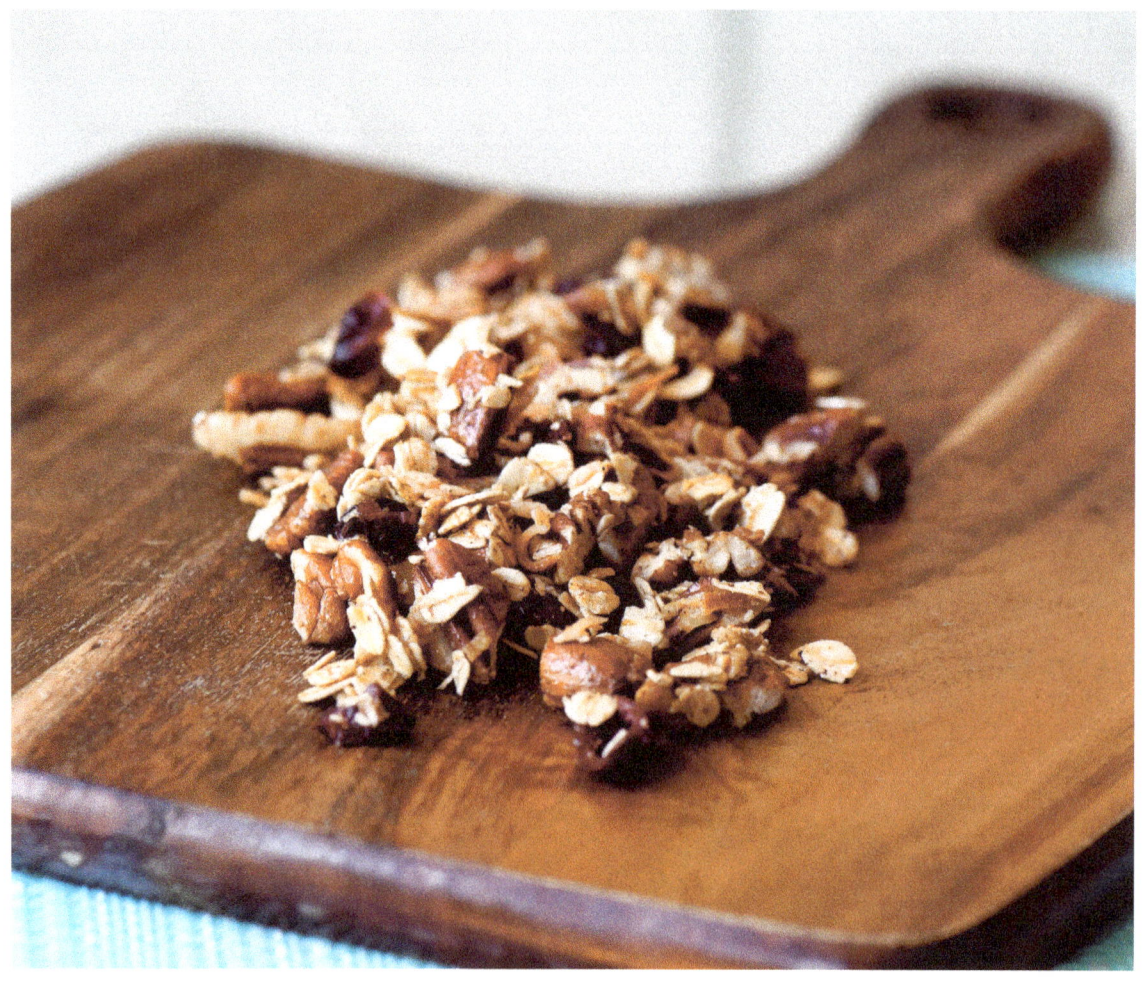

Prep Time: 20 mins | Total Time: 30 minutes | Serves: 8 cups

WHAT YOU'LL NEED:

1 ½ cups pecan pieces

1 cup dried cranberries

1 ½ tsp. cinnamon

2 tbsp. pure maple syrup

4 cup rolled oats

1 cup of almonds

2 tsp. vanilla essence

⅓ tsp. nutmeg

1 cup unsweetened coconut flakes

Almond or coconut milk, to serve

WHAT TO DO:

- Preheat oven to 180 degrees.

- Put the oats onto a sheet of baking paper and then sprinkle the coconut on top. Put the pecan pieces on a second sheet of baking paper. Bake both for around 10 minutes until the coconut is golden brown. Take them out of the oven and allow to cool.

- In a small bowl combine the vanilla essence and maple syrup. Warm for 20 seconds in a microwave.

- In a large bowl add the cranberries, toasted pecans, oats, coconut, maple mixture and the spices. Stir to combine. Transfer this mixture onto a sheet of baking paper. Spread to an even layer. Let the mixture dry for about 10 minutes. Break up and store in an air tight container

- Add your choice of milk to serve.

Mushroom and Spinach Omelette

Get your taste buds ready for this delicious and healthy breakfast, lunch or dinner.

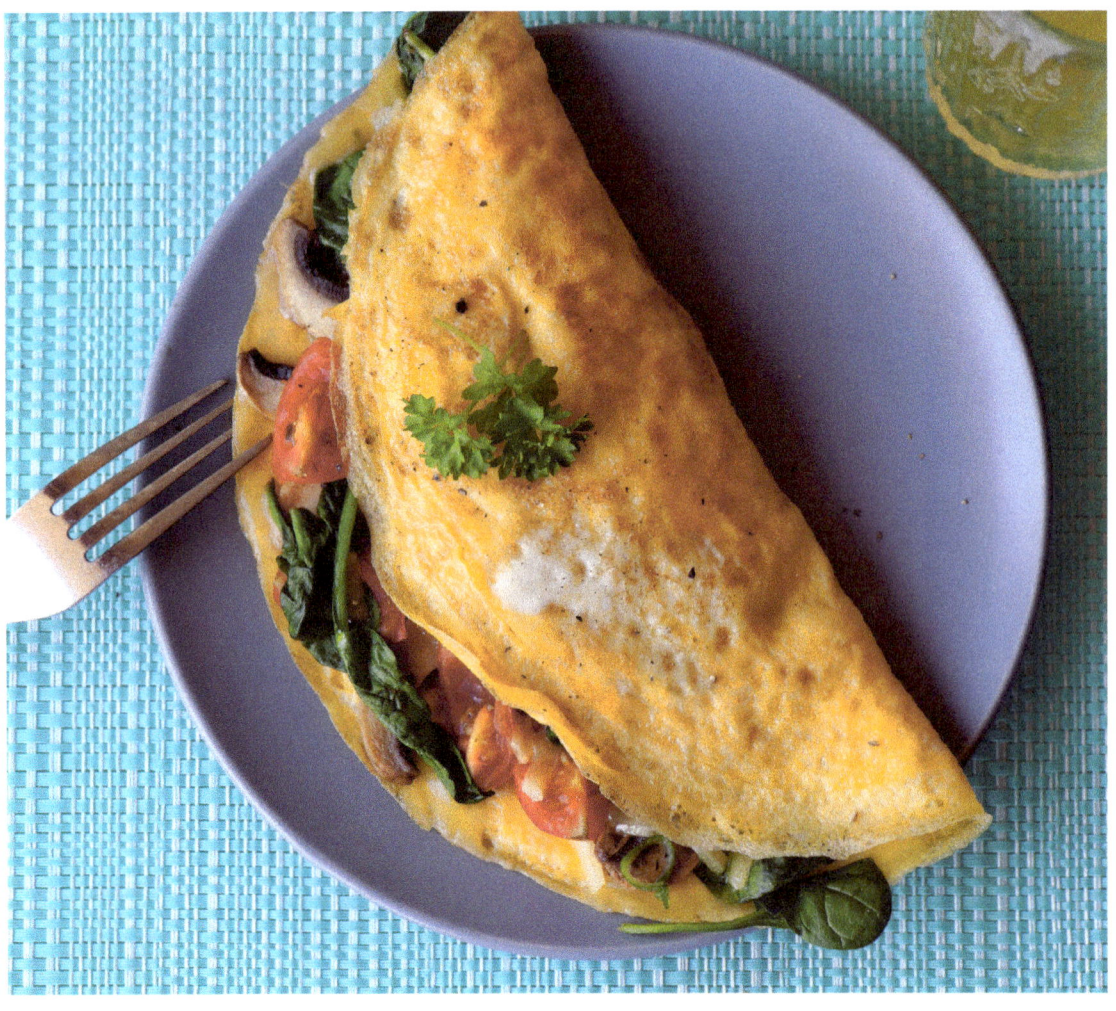

Prep Time: 5 mins | Total Time: 20 mins | Serves: 1

WHAT YOU'LL NEED:

3 eggs

1 cup mushrooms (sliced)

1 cup baby spinach

½ cup of cherry tomatoes (quartered)

½ spring onion (sliced)

⅓ cup of grated cheese

Olive oil spray

Salt and pepper, to taste

2 tbsp. cheese (grated)

Chopped fresh parsley (to garnish)

WHAT TO DO:

- Spray a non-stick pan with olive oil and place over a medium heat. Add in the mushrooms, tomatoes and spring onions and cook for 5-6 minutes. Add in spinach and take them off the heat and transfer to a bowl.

- Use a paper towel to clean the pan, spray with olive oil and heat up the pan again.

- Whisk together the eggs with salt and black pepper in a small bowl. Pour the eggs into the pan and cook for 6-7 minutes, until the edges have set.

- Layer half of it with mushrooms, tomatoes, onions, spinach and cheese. Fold half the omelette over the veggies.

- Transfer to a plate. Garnish with parley and serve.

Baked Beans

Quick, easy, and so much tastier than their canned cousins.

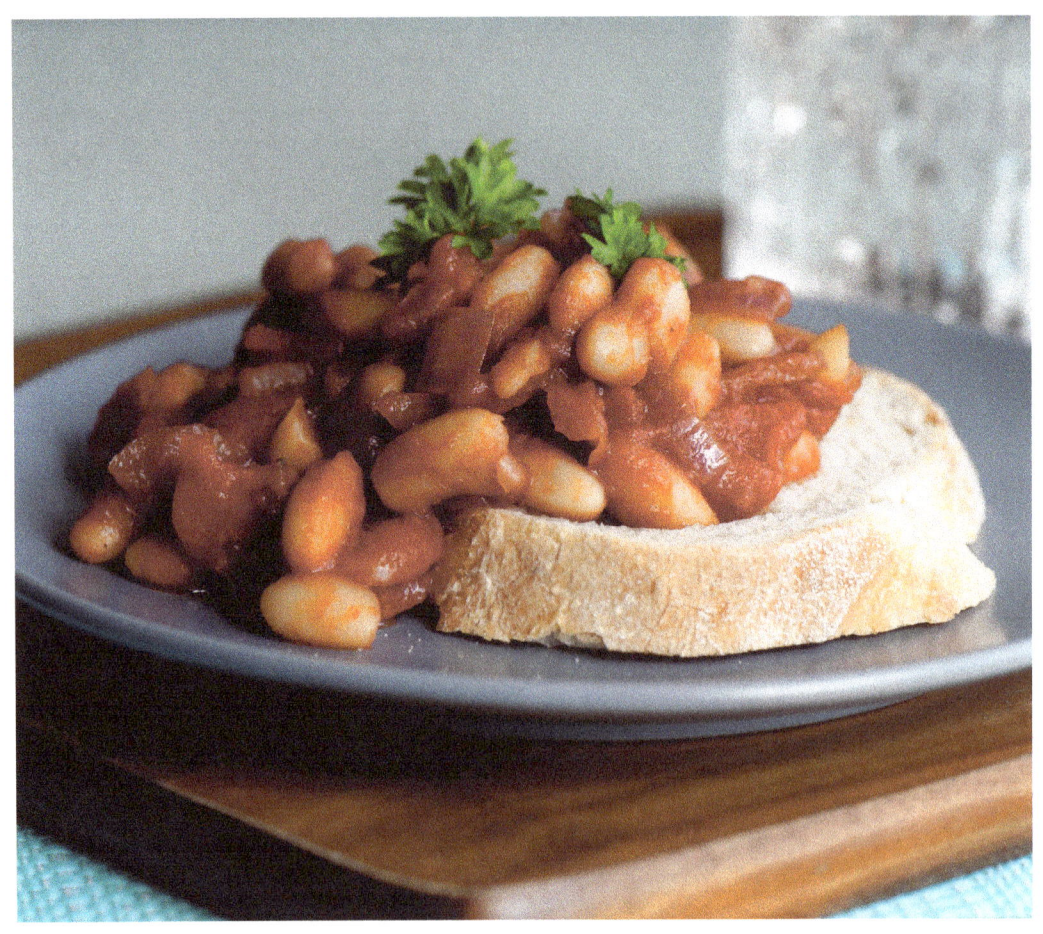

Prep Time: 2 mins | Total Time: 15mins | Serves 2

WHAT YOU'LL NEED:

2 cups of Cannelloni beans

1 can of tinned tomatoes

2 tbsp. of tomato paste

½ a red onion

Parsley to garnish

WHAT TO DO:

- Soak the Cannelloni beans overnight.

- Drain and rinse the beans.

- Chop and fry the onion until browned.

- Add beans, tinned tomatoes and tomato paste to pan.

- Allow to simmer for 10 minutes until liquid has reduced.

- Serve on a slice of toast. Sprinkle with cracked black pepper to taste, and garnish with parley.

Roasted Tomato Soup

This soup is packed full of flavour and you'll be wanting to make this on every chilly night to enjoy some warm comfort food.

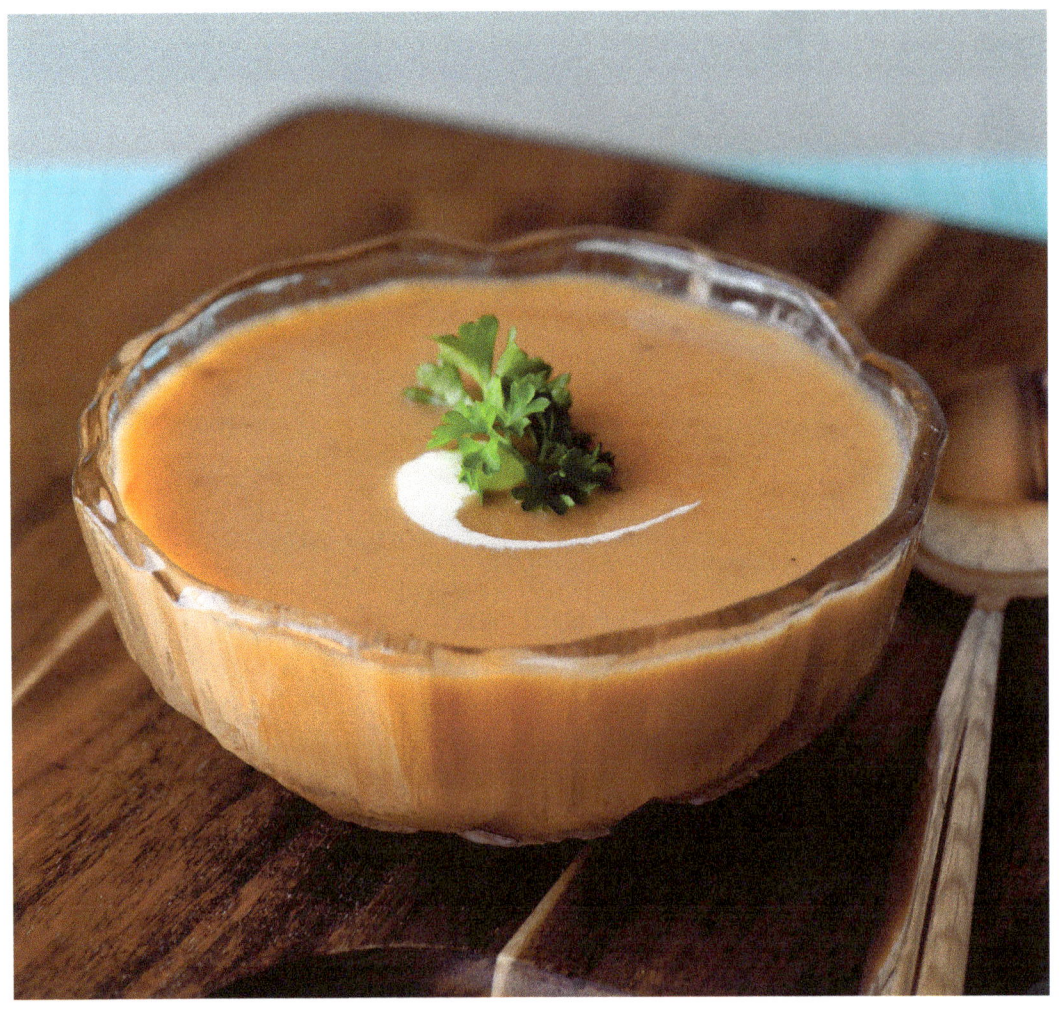

Prep Time: 10 minutes | Total Time: 55 minutes | Serves: 4

WHAT YOU'LL NEED:

1 kg of ripe tomatoes

3 cups chicken stock

2 tsp. fresh parsley

2 tbsp. balsamic vinegar

1 garlic clove (minced)

2 tbsp. olive oil

1 onion (chopped)

¼ cup cream

½ cup dry white wine

Salt and black pepper, to taste

Parsley, to garnish

WHAT TO DO:

- Preheat oven to 180 degrees.

- To roast the tomatoes: Slice the tomatoes in half and place on a sheet of baking paper with the cut side up. In a small bowl, whisk the vinegar, half the olive oil, parsley, minced garlic, salt and pepper together. Drizzle this mixture over the tomatoes and place them in the oven for 20-30 minutes or until soft.

- To make the soup: Place a large soup pot over a medium heat. Heat the remaining olive oil in the pot. Add in the chopped onion fry until browned. Add the white wine and bring mixture to a boil. Cook for around 5 minutes or until liquid is evaporated. Pour in the chicken stock and the roasted tomatoes. Bring to a boil. Reduce the heat and let it simmer for 10 minutes.

- Allow the soup to cool down and then puree it using a stick blender or regular blender. Return to heat and allow to simmer for a few minutes.

- Before serving, stir in the cream, then add garnish.

Asian Style Meatballs

These meatballs are packed full of the flavours of Asian
cooking that we all love.

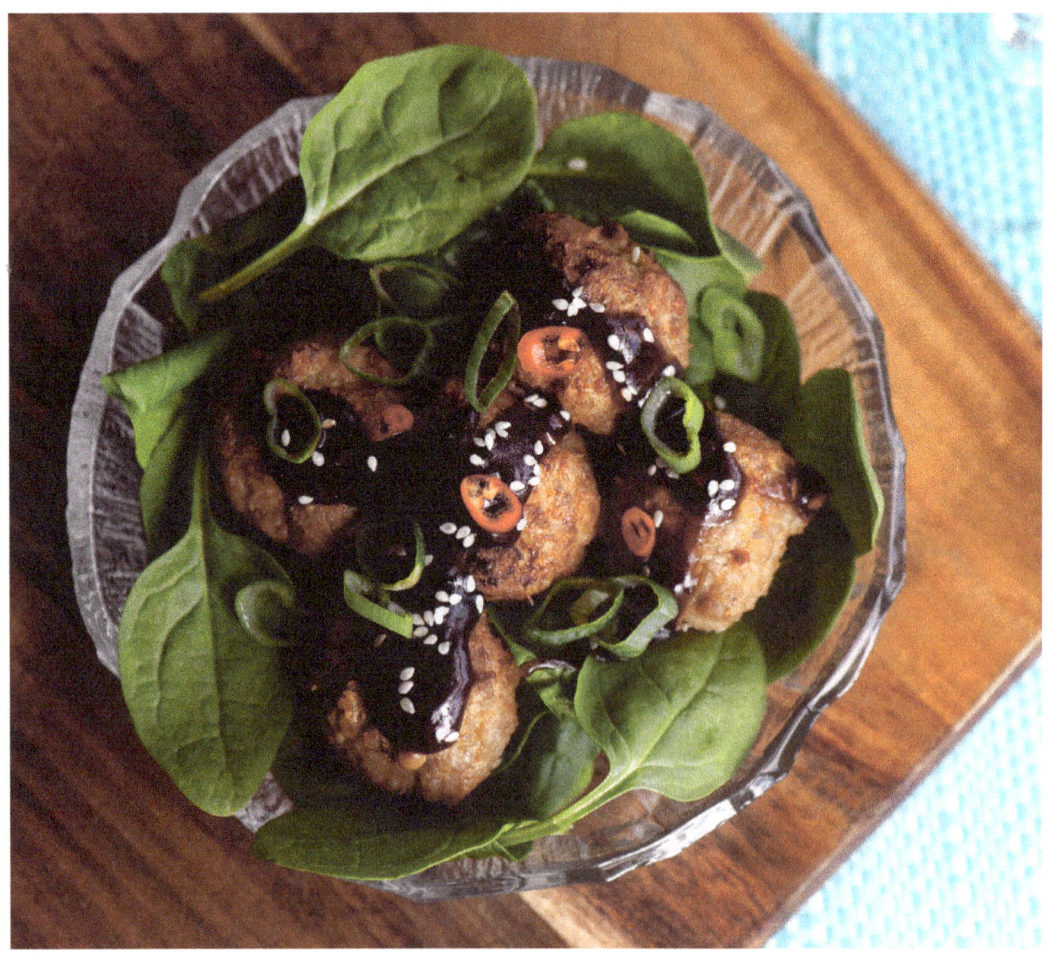

Prep Time: 15 mins | Total Time: 35 mins | Serves: 20 meatballs

WHAT YOU'LL NEED:

500g turkey mince

1 large egg

2 tsp. sesame oil

¾ cup cooked quinoa

½ tsp. cayenne pepper

3 garlic cloves (minced)

1 tbsp. soy sauce

2 spring onions (thinly sliced)

FOR THE SAUCE:

1 tsp. sesame oil

2 tbsp. rice vinegar

2 tsp. cornflour

¼ cup soy sauce

1 tbsp. brown sugar

½ tsp. cayenne pepper

1 tbsp. freshly grated ginger

½ tsp. sesame seeds

WHAT TO DO:

- Preheat oven to 180 degrees. Line a baking tray with a sheet of baking paper.

- In a large bowl, combine the quinoa, egg, turkey, sesame oil, onions, garlic, cayenne pepper, soy sauce, salt and pepper in a large bowl. Mix everything together. Make around 18-20 meatballs from the mixture and place them on the prepared baking tray. Bake for 20 minutes or until cooked and browned on top.

- Place a small saucepan over a medium heat. Add the sugar, soy sauce, ginger, sesame oil, rice vinegar and ½ cup water to make the sauce.

- In a small bowl whisk the cornflour and 1 tbsp. water together and pour this mixture into the pan with the sauce. Simmer for 2 minutes, until thickened.

- Serve the meatballs with the sauce and garnish with sesame seeds and spring onions.

Toast Stack

Silky and smooth avocado topped with some scrambled eggs and salsa.

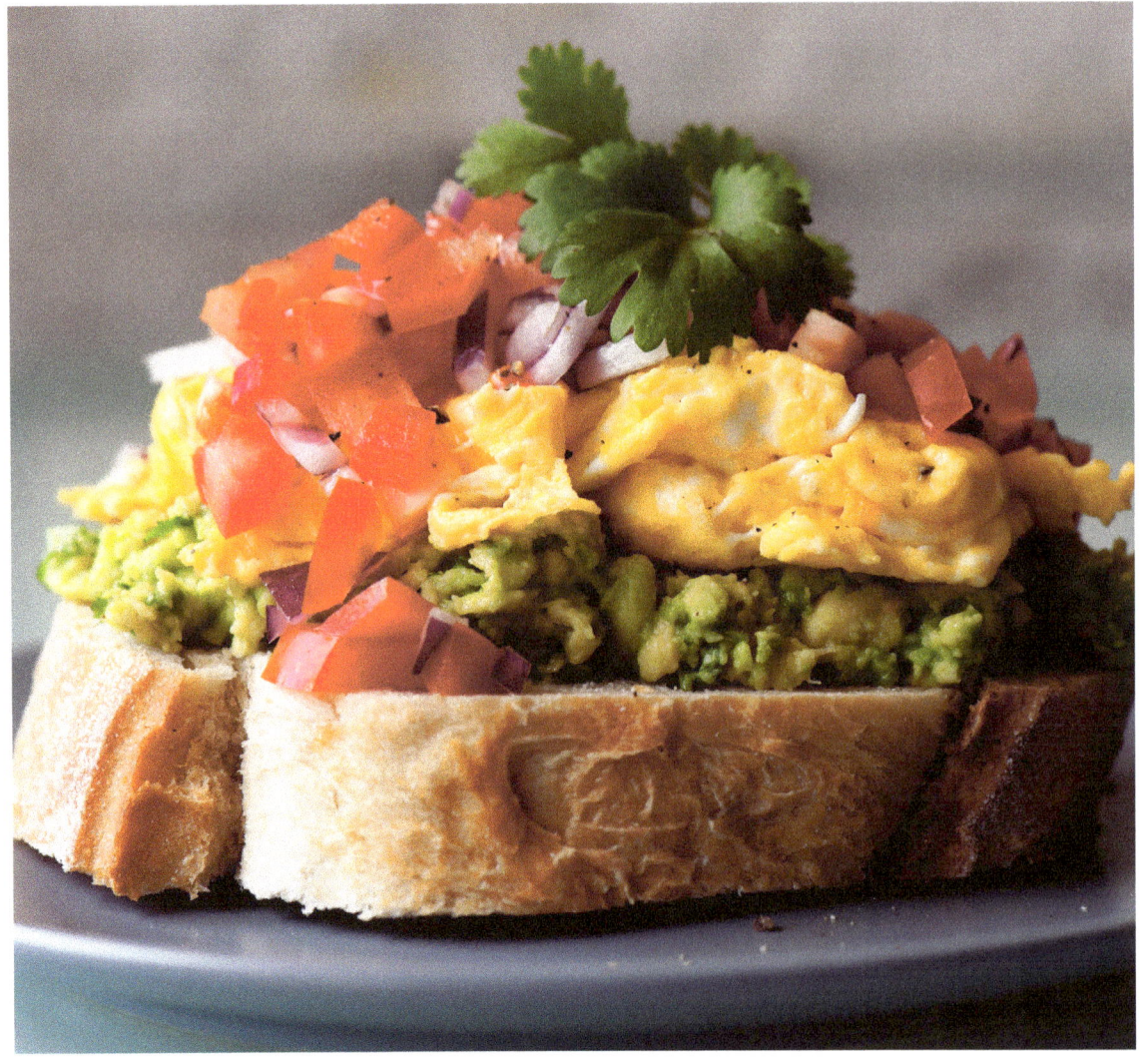

Prep Time: 10 mins | Total Time: 15 mins | Serves: 2

WHAT YOU'LL NEED:

1 avocado (peeled and seeded)

4 eggs

Juice of ½ lime

2 tsp. coriander

4 slices of toast

Salt and pepper

FOR THE SALSA:

1 roma tomato

¼ a red onion

¼ a red capsicum

½ a chilli

WHAT TO DO:

- Mix avocado, lime, and coriander in a bowl. Stir until mashed.

- Spread the mixture on the pieces of toast.

- Prepare salsa by finely chopping all ingredients and mixing in a small bowl.

- Whisk eggs, salt and pepper together in a small bowl.
  Spray a non-stick pan with olive oil and place over a low heat.
  Add the eggs and scramble them until cooked.
  Place scrambled egg on top of the avocado mash.

- Place salsa on top.

- Garnish with coriander and serve.

Zucchini Side Dish

An unusual side dish that will be a hit with guests.

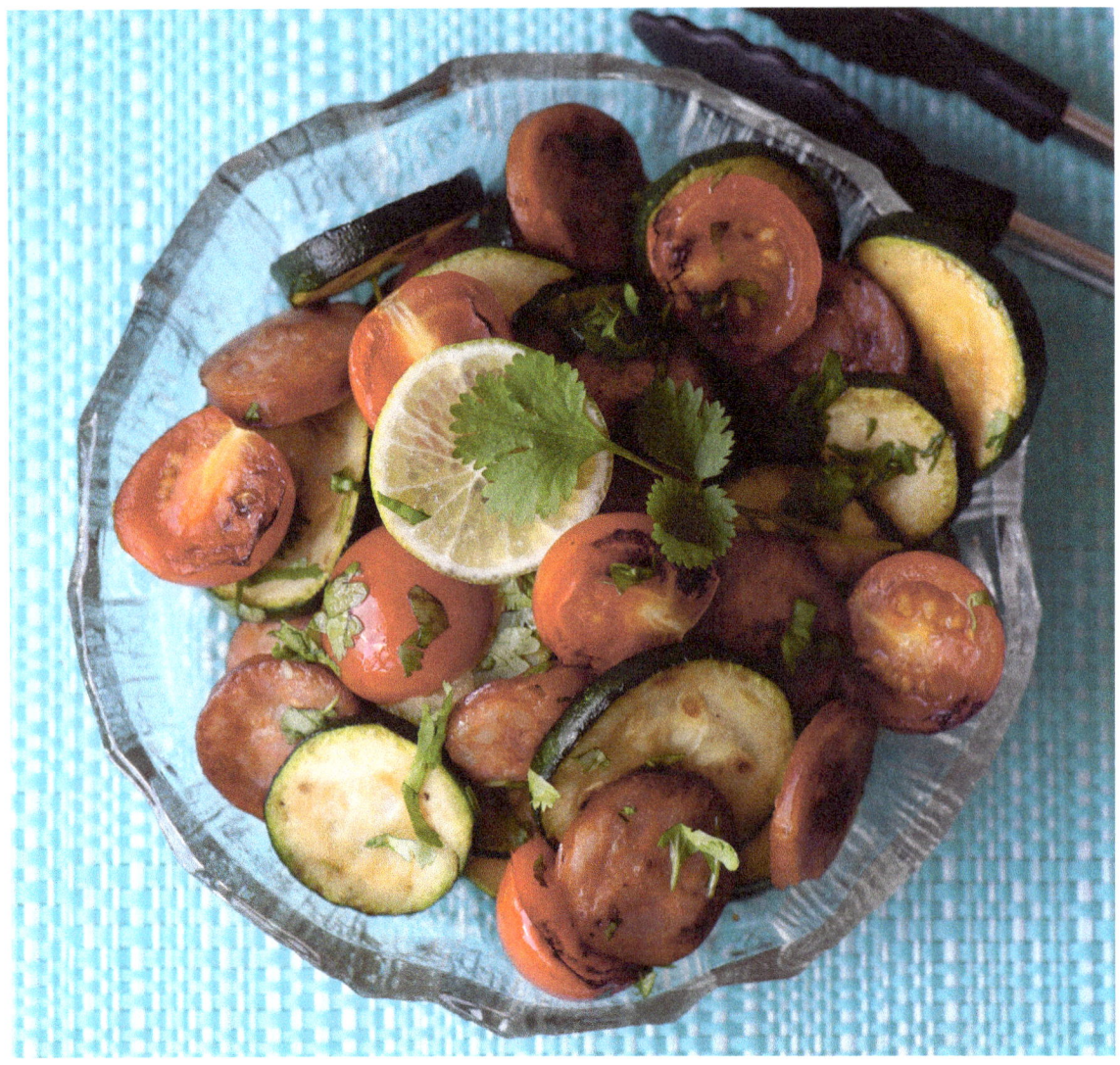

Prep Time: 10 mins | Total Time: 25 mins | Serves: 4

WHAT YOU'LL NEED:

3 medium zucchini

1 Spanish chorizo

1 lime

1 cup of cherry tomatoes

½ cup coriander (roughly chopped)

Olive oil spray

Salt to taste

WHAT TO DO:

- Slice the zucchini and chorizo and halve the cherry tomatoes. Zest and juice the lime. Set all aside.

- Place a large pan over a medium heat and spray with olive oil. Add the chorizo and cook for 5 minutes, until slightly crispy. Transfer to a plate and set aside.

- In the same pan, add the zucchini and turn the heat up slightly. Occasionally toss the zucchini for 10 minutes or until cooked. Add in the tomatoes until slightly cooked.

- Add in the lime zest, lime juice, chorizo and coriander.

- Season with salt and serve.

Egg Filled Mushroom Cups

This makes for a fun breakfast, an easy lunch option or
even serves as a snack.

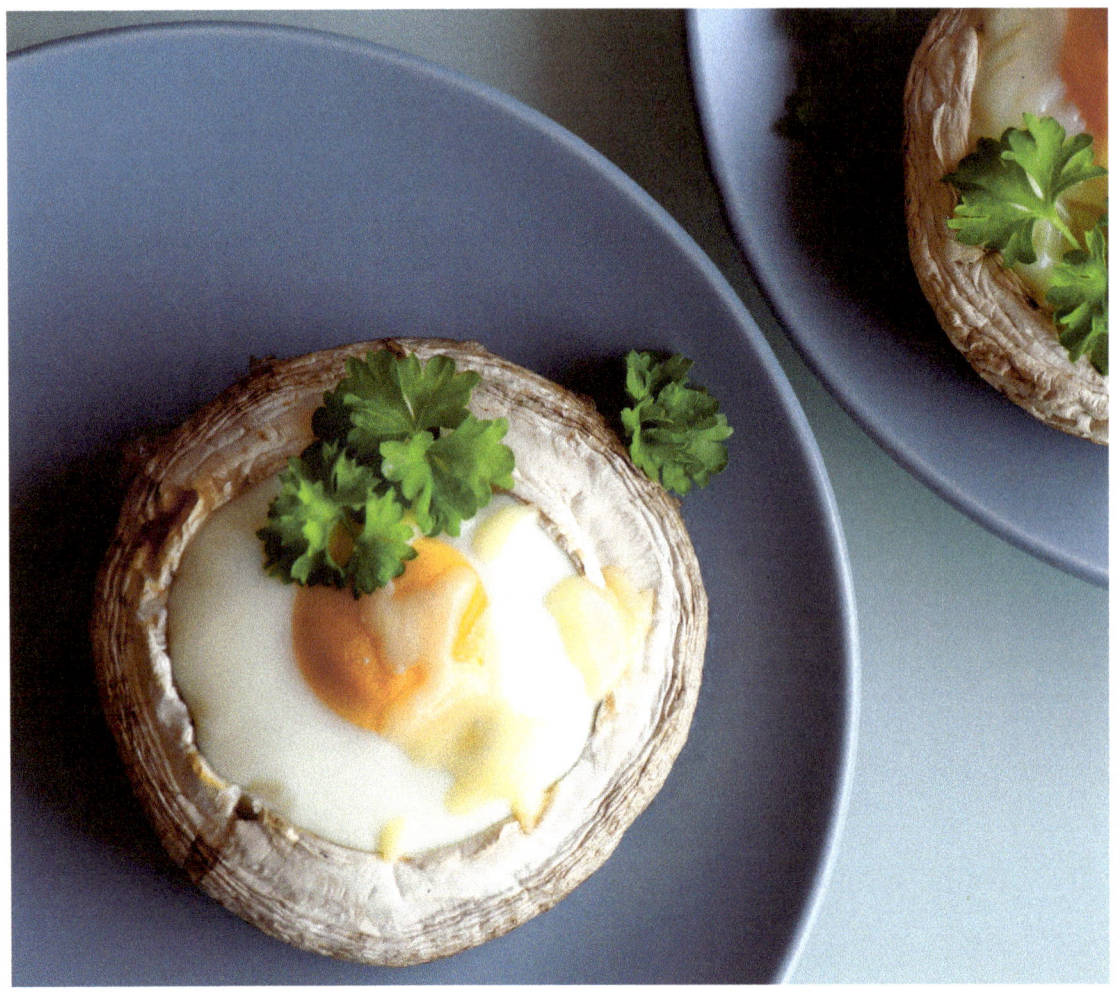

Prep Time: 5 mins | Total Time: 30 mins | Serves: 2

WHAT YOU'LL NEED:

4 large eggs

4 large mushrooms

½ cup shaved Parmesan cheese

Olive oil spray

Salt and pepper

Parsley to garnish

WHAT TO DO:

- Preheat oven to 180 degrees.

- Wash and take the stalks out of the mushrooms. Pat them dry with paper towels and spray with olive oil cooking spray on both sides.

- Crack an egg into each mushroom. Place in the oven on a tray lined with a sheet of baking paper.

- Bake for 20 minutes or until egg has set. Sprinkle with cheese and bake for another 5 minutes until cheese has melted.

- Season with the salt and pepper to taste. Garnish with parsley.

Chicken and Quinoa Casserole

Healthy and creamy farmhouse style casserole.

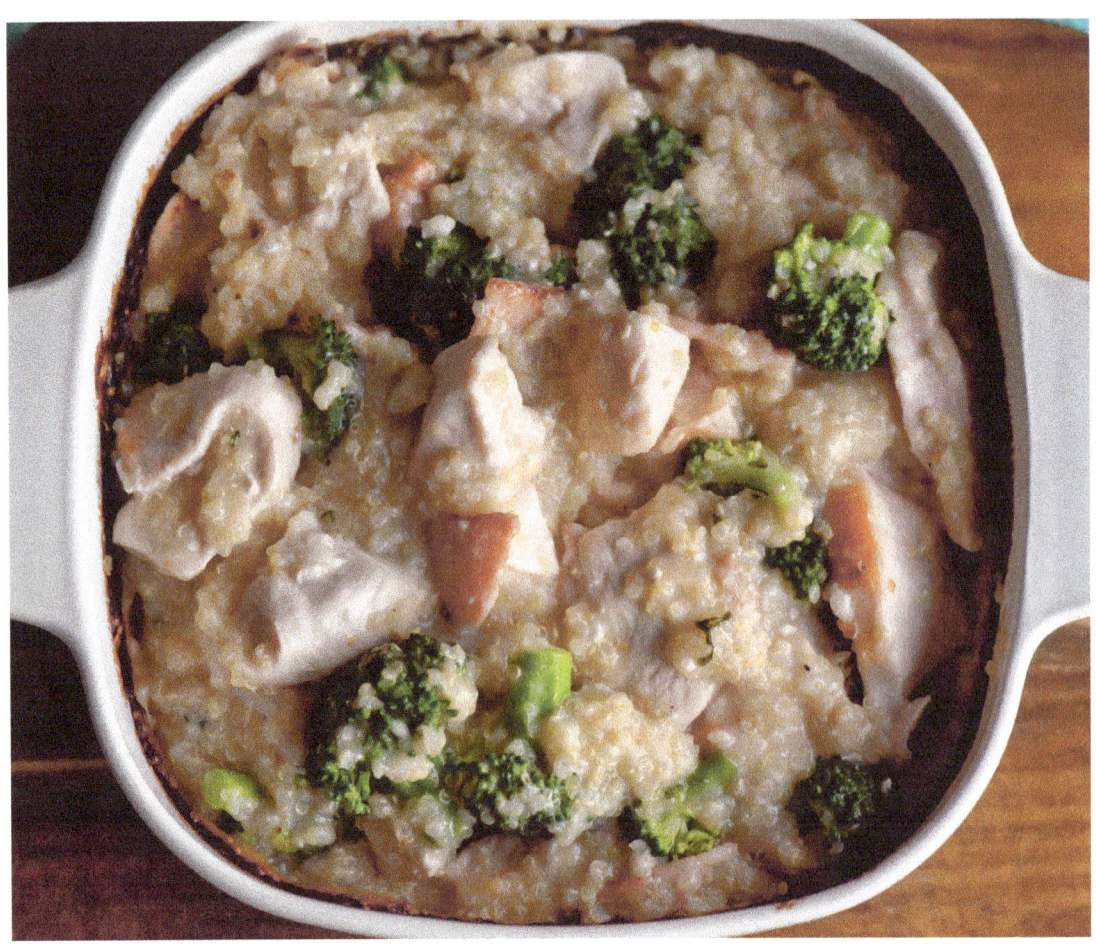

Prep Time: 15 mins | Total Time: 1 hour 15 mins | Serves: 6

WHAT YOU'LL NEED:

1kg chicken breasts
(cut into pieces)

1 cup uncooked quinoa (rinsed)

1 cup milk

¼ cup cooked bacon

2 cups fresh broccoli florets

½ tsp. cayenne pepper

½ cup flour

2 cups chicken stock

1 tsp. all purpose seasoning

2 cups water

1 tsp. mixed herbs

Olive oil spray

WHAT TO DO:

- Preheat oven to 180 degrees and grease a baking dish with olive oil spray.

- In a saucepan, bring ½ cup milk and chicken stock to a boil. Whisk the remaining ½ cup milk with the flour, cayenne pepper, seasoning and herbs. Add this mixture into the saucepan and whisk until it makes a creamy sauce. Add 1 cup water, bacon and quinoa to the saucepan and stir to combine. Transfer this mixture into the prepared baking dish and top with chicken breasts pieces. Bake for 30 minutes.

- In a small saucepan, boil the broccoli for 1 minute and set aside.

- Stir the casserole after 30 minutes, then bake for a further 10 minutes. Once the chicken and quinoa has cooked, stir the broccoli and add a bit of water, if needed. Bake for a further 5 minutes.

- (Optional - Sprinkle cheese on top and bake until the cheese is melted.)

Grilled Salmon with Avocado

A tasty and refreshing avocado salsa tops this off. Perfect for any meal of the day.

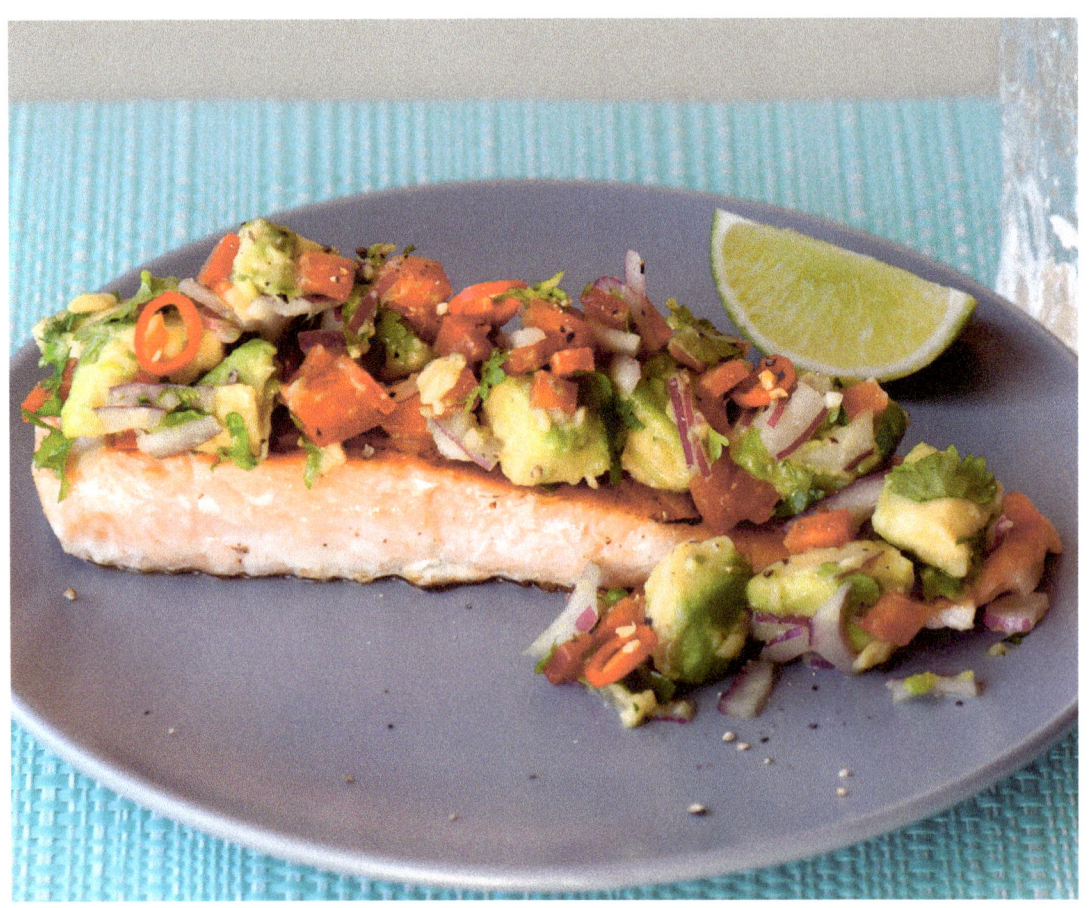

Prep Time: 15 mins | Total Time: 25 mins | Serves: 4

WHAT YOU'LL NEED:

1 tsp. ground cumin

4 salmon fillets

1 tbsp. olive oil

Salt and freshly ground black pepper, to taste

Olive oil spray

FOR THE AVOCADO SALSA:

1 small avocado (diced)

1 tbsp. fresh lemon juice

¼ cup fresh parsley (chopped)

¼ cup capsicum (diced)

¼ cup red onion (diced)

1 ½ tsp. garlic (minced)

½ a chilli (sliced)

2 tbsp. fresh coriander (chopped)

2 tbsp. rice wine vinegar

3 tbsp. olive oil

WHAT TO DO:

- Place a pan over medium heat. Brush both sides of the salmon with 1 tbsp. olive oil and season with cumin, salt, and pepper.

- Spray the pan with olive oil and cook the fish for 3-4 minutes on each side, until salmon is cooked.

- Make the salsa by combining all ingredients in a small bowl.

- Top the salmon with the avocado salsa and serve.

- (Optional - serve on a bed of brown rice or with a garden salad.)

Thai Stir Fry

This vegetarian style Thai stir fry is super easy to put together and makes for a delicious lunch or dinner for days when you don't have much time on your hands.

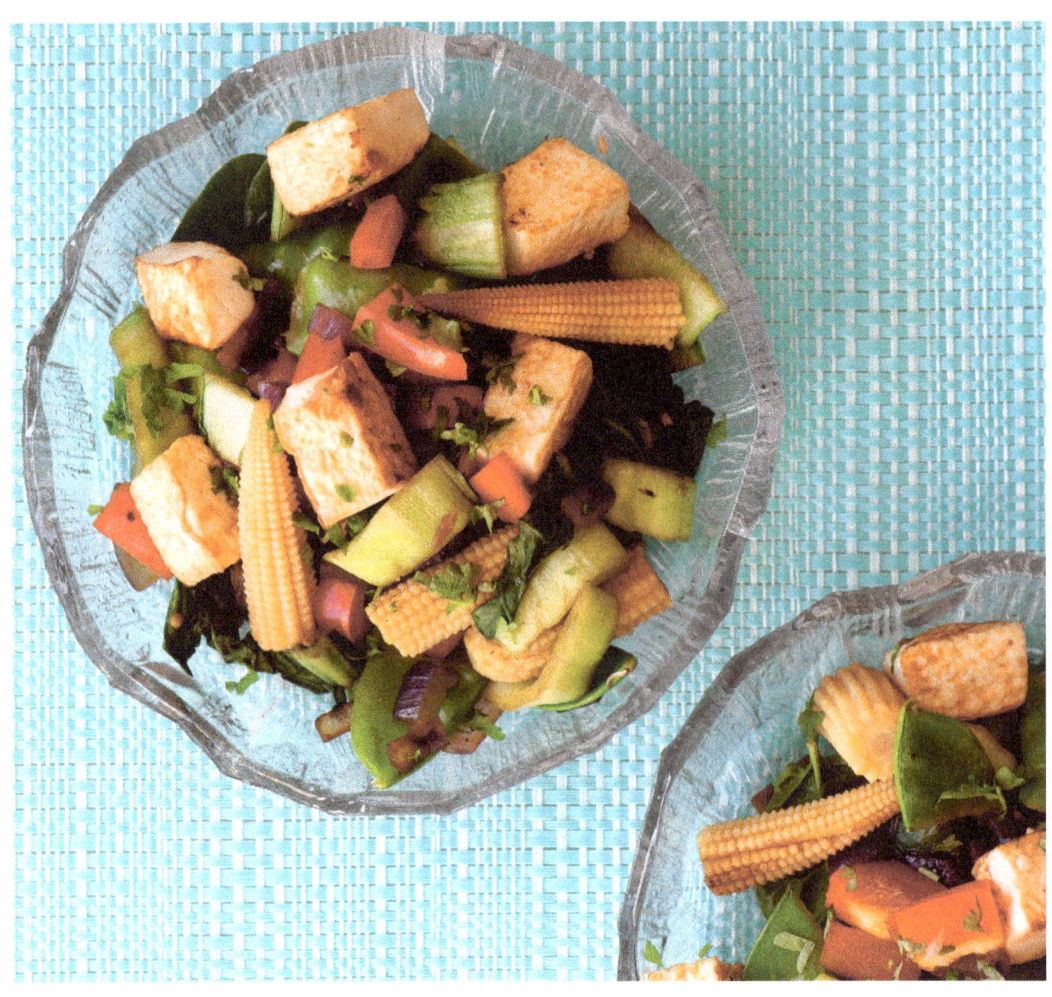

Prep Time: 10 mins | Total Time: 20 mins | Serves: 4

WHAT YOU'LL NEED:

1 packet of tofu, diced

1 capsicum (diced)

1 tbsp. coconut oil

2cm piece of ginger (grated)

1 cup snow peas
(roughly chopped)

1 cup of bok choi (chopped)

1 onion (diced)

¼ cup basil (chopped roughly)

1 cup baby corn

½ lime (zest and juice)

1 tbsp. soy sauce

WHAT TO DO:

- Place pan over a medium heat. Add the coconut oil. Add the ginger and onion and cook until onion starts to soften. Set aside.

- In the same pan, fry the tofu until is browned on all sides.

- Re-add the onion and ginger mix. Then add the corn, capsicum, and snow peas. Continue cooking this on medium heat for around 10 minutes, until everything is hot and starts to turn golden.

- Add in the bok choi, along with the soy sauce, lime juice, lime zest and basil.

- Stir everything together and serve.

Balsamic Chicken with Vegetables

One pan is all you'll need for this simple meal that will be a
hit with the whole family.

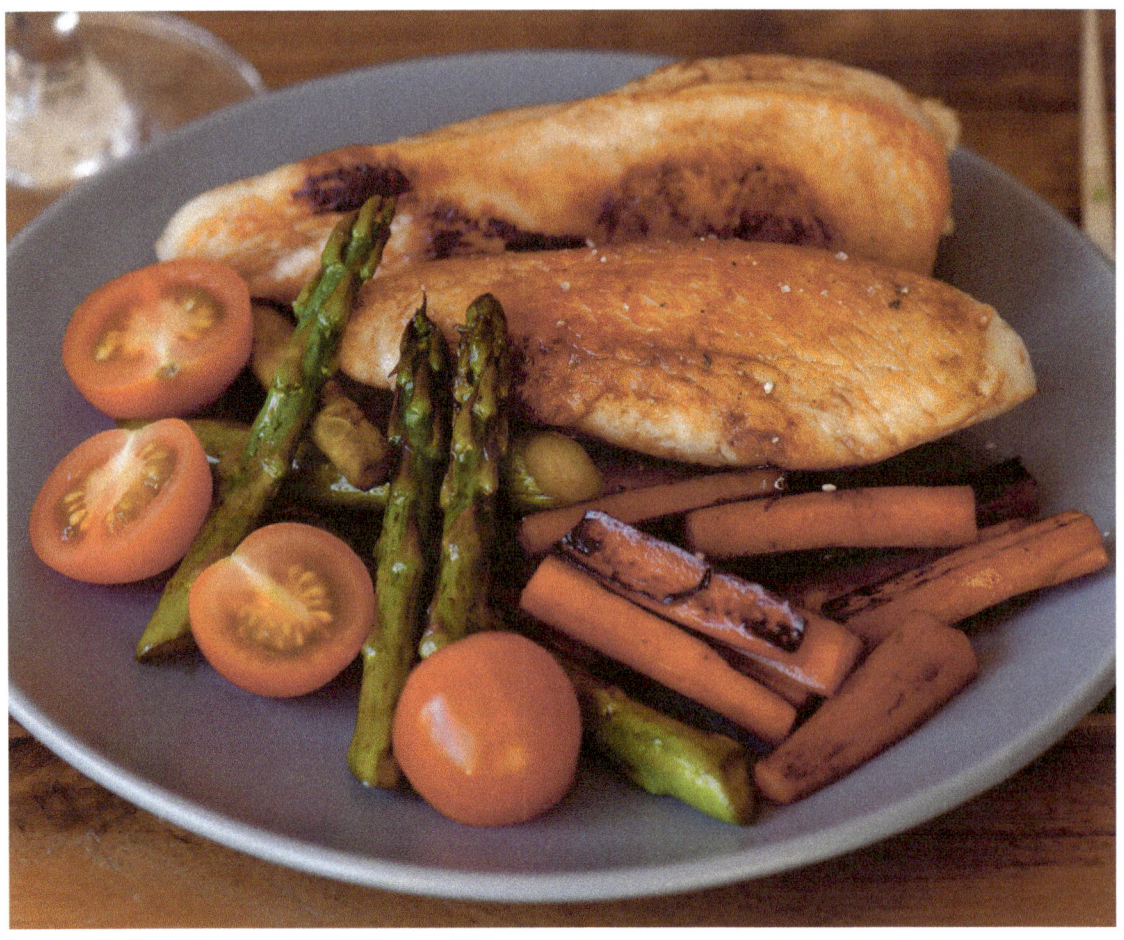

Prep Time: 10 mins | Total Time: 23 mins | Serves: 4

WHAT YOU'LL NEED:

1 kg chicken breast

1 ½ tbsp. honey

2 tbsp. olive oil

1 bunch fresh asparagus
(chopped into 5cm pieces)

3 tbsp. balsamic vinegar

1 ½ cups carrots (cut into matchsticks)

Dash of tabasco sauce

1 cup cherry tomatoes (halved)

Salt and black pepper, to taste

WHAT TO DO:

- In a small bowl whisk the honey, vinegar and tabasco together. Set aside.

- Place a medium pan over medium-high heat and add olive oil. Season the chicken breasts with salt and pepper and cook for 3-4 minutes on each side, until cooked through.
  Whilst the chicken is cooking, chop up the vegetables.

- Add half of the dressing into the pan and coat the chicken with it. Transfer to a plate and set aside.

- In the same pan add the carrots and asparagus and season with salt and pepper. Stir everything together and cook for around 5 minutes. Transfer the veggies onto a serving plate with the chicken.

- Pour the remaining dressing into the pan and cook while stirring for a minute or two until thickened.

- Add the fresh tomatoes to the serving plate and drizzle the dressing on top. Serve.

Kale and Sweet Potato Curry

This is a one pot curry that just screams comfort food.
A creamy curry, with a flavour that packs a punch.

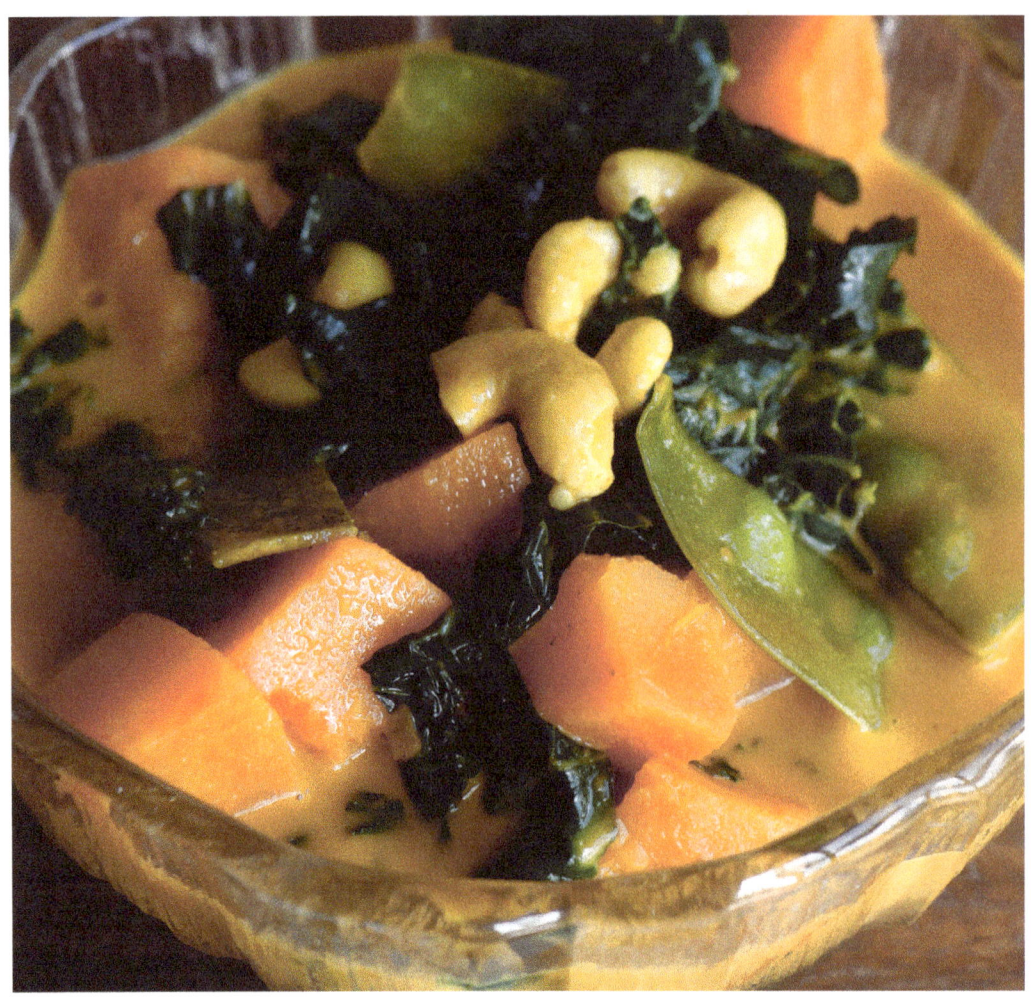

Prep Time: 5 mins | Total Time: 30 mins | Serves: 2-4

WHAT YOU'LL NEED:

1 large sweet potato (peeled and cubed)

1 tbsp. honey

1 lemon, juiced

1 ½ tbsp. coconut oil

3 tbsp. red curry paste

2 tbsp. fresh ginger (minced)

2 cups chopped kale

1 cup snow peas

2 cans light coconut milk

2 tbsp. minced garlic

½ cup roasted cashews

1 ½ tsp. ground turmeric

Salt to taste

WHAT TO DO:

- Place a large pot over medium heat. Once it heats up, add in coconut oil, garlic and ginger. Cook for two minutes while stirring.

- Add in the sweet potato and red curry paste. Cook for 2 minutes while stirring.

- Add in coconut milk, turmeric, and honey. Stir and bring to a simmer. Once mixture starts simmering, add peas and reduce heat slightly.

- Cook for 5-10 minutes, stirring occasionally until the potatoes and peas soften.

- Add in cashews, lemon juice and kale. Cover and let it simmer for 3-4 minutes over medium-low heat.

- Serve.

Avocado and Ricotta Fritters

These fritters sure taste amazing for an avocado lover.

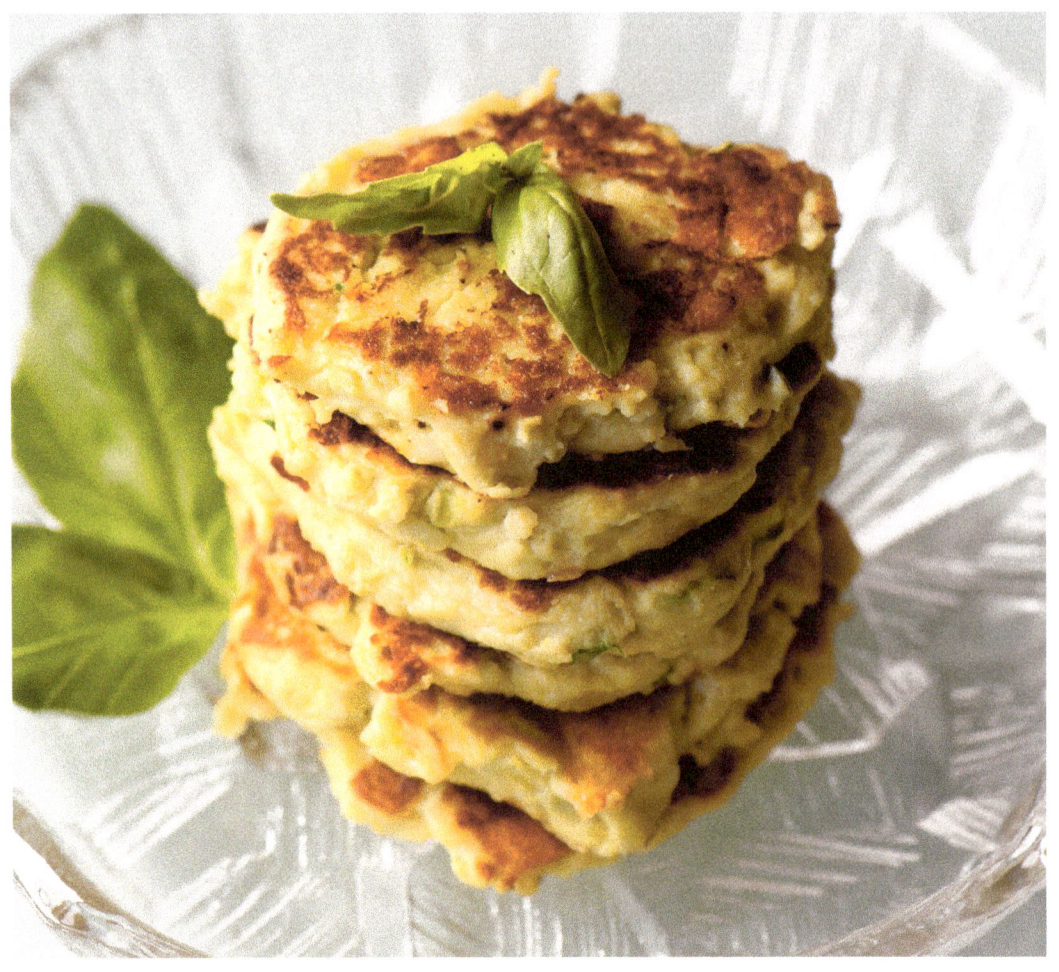

Prep Time: 5 minutes | Total Time: 20 minutes | Serves: 2

WHAT YOU'LL NEED:

1 egg

200 grams ricotta

Salt and pepper

Juice of ½ lime

1 ripe avocado (mashed)

½ a cup of flour
(or substitute almond meal)

A few basil leaves

½ cup finely shredded
Parmesan cheese

1 tbsp. olive oil

WHAT TO DO:

- In a small bowl, whisk the egg and add in salt and pepper.

- Place a large pan over a medium heat. Heat olive oil in pan.

- In a large bowl, combine the egg with the flour and mix well until texture is smooth. Add the ricotta and avocado and stir until combined. Add the cheese, finely chopped basil leaves and lime juice. Stir until well combined.

- Take a large spoonful of the mix and place it in the pan, flattening slightly into a fritter shape. Place a few in the pan at once, without crowding. Fry until both sides turn light golden. Repeat until all mix has been cooked.

- Serve hot.

Grilled Chicken with Pesto

A healthy and tasty chicken recipe that's topped with pesto and cheese.

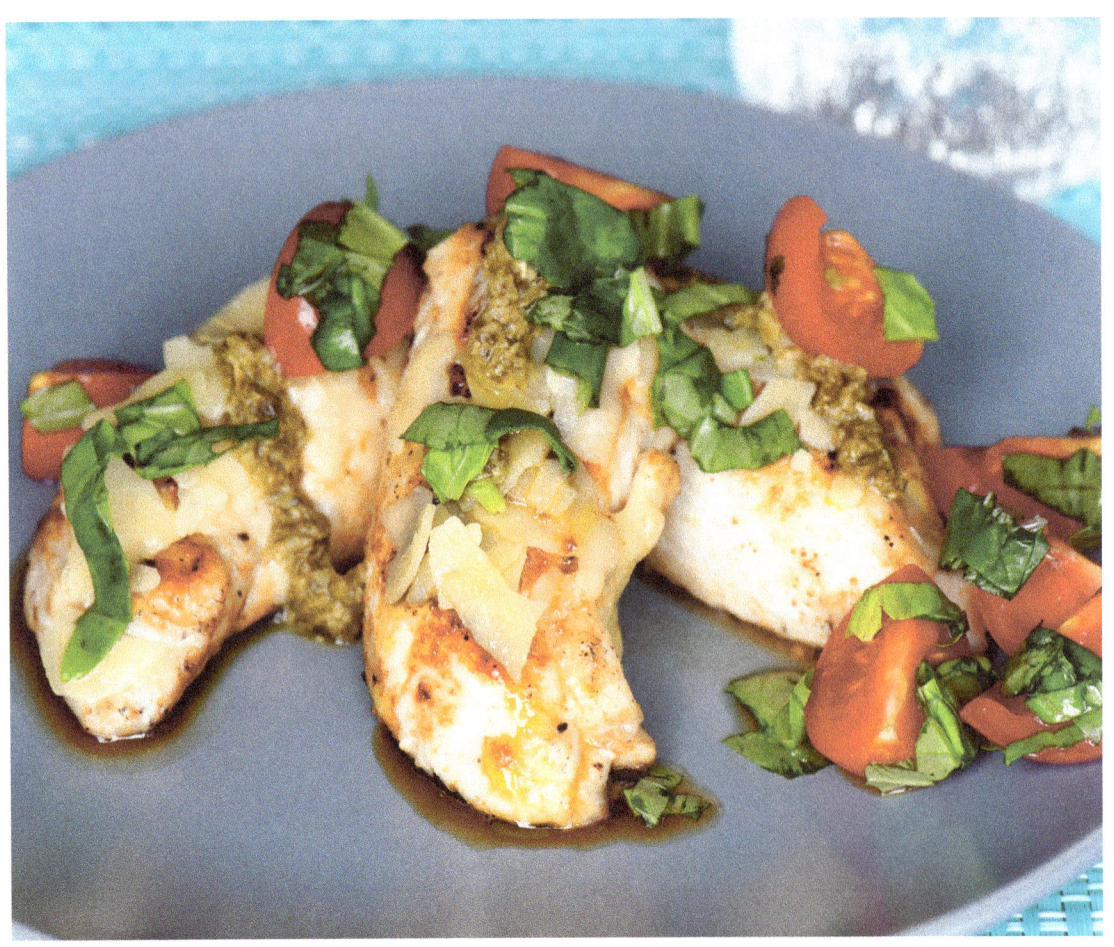

Prep Time: 10 mins | Total Time: 30 mins | Serves: 4

WHAT YOU'LL NEED:

4 chicken breasts

2 tbsp. olive oil

½ cup cherry tomatoes (quartered)

1 tsp. all purpose seasoning

1 tbsp. fresh lemon juice

1 tsp. garlic powder

½ cup basil pesto

¼ cup basil leaves (chopped)

¼ cup shaved parmesan cheese

Black pepper, to taste

Salt, to taste

WHAT TO DO:

- Combine the chicken, olive oil, seasoning, garlic powder, salt and pepper together in a large bowl.

- Grill the chicken in a grill pan over medium-high heat for around 6-8 minutes on each side or until cooked. Place cheese on top of the chicken while it is still in the pan. Cook for 1 more minute to the cheese melts slightly.

- Toss the basil, tomatoes and lemon juice together in a small bowl.

- Top the chicken with a scoop of tomatoes, 3 tbsp. pesto and some freshly cracked pepper.

- Serve.

Sticky Beef Strips

This dinner will be on your table in 30 minutes and tastes oh so yummy!

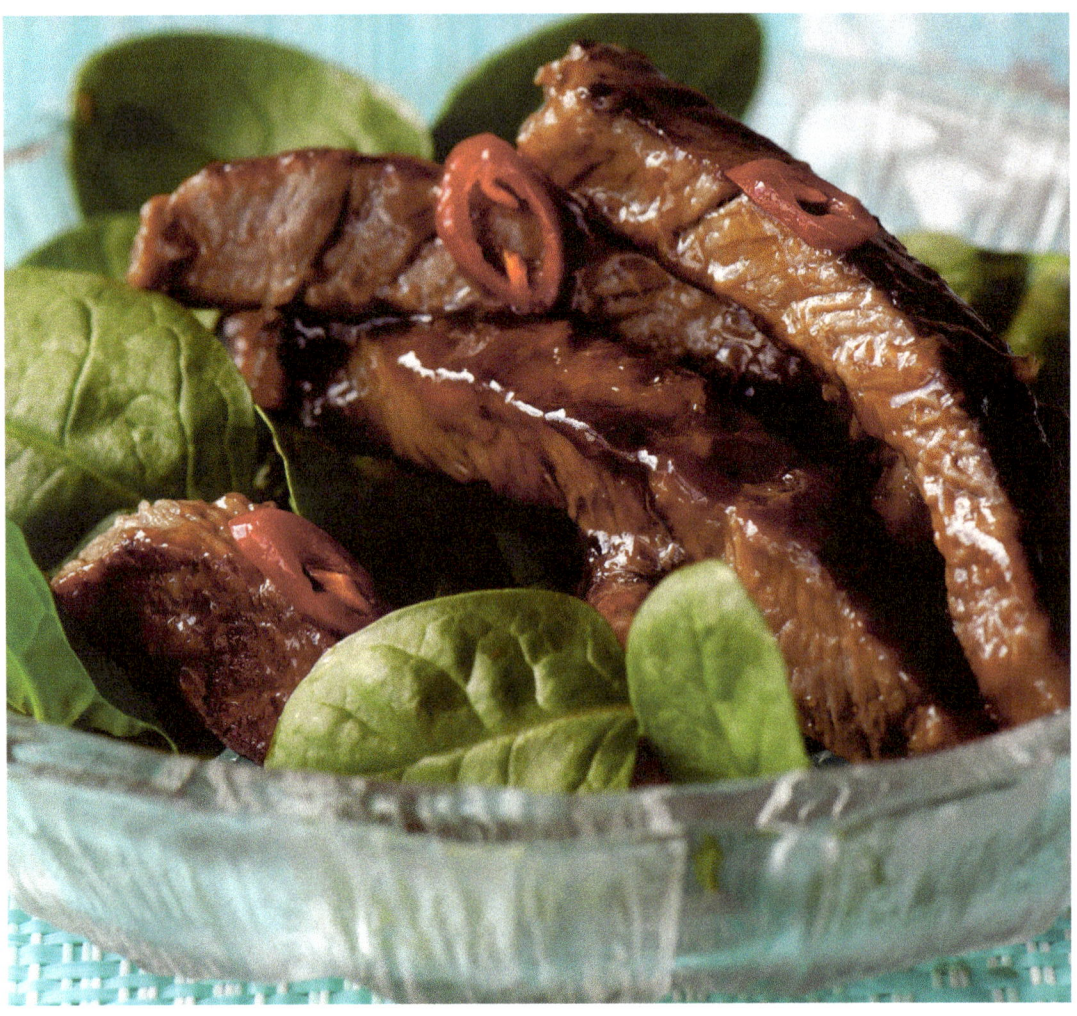

Prep Time: 15 minutes | Total Time: 30 minutes | Serves: 4

WHAT YOU'LL NEED:

1 kg sirloin steak (sliced thinly)

1 tbsp. olive oil

¼ cup soy sauce

2 tbsp. + 1 tbsp. cornflour

1 tbsp. Worcestershire sauce

1 tbsp. fresh ginger (grated)

½ cup beef stock

¼ cup pure maple syrup
(or substitute honey)

1 pinch chilli powder

2 tsp. garlic (minced)

Optional - ½ chilli (sliced)

WHAT TO DO:

- Toss the beef steak with 2 tbsp. cornflour and let it sit for 2-3 minutes.

- Add oil to a large pan over high heat. Once the oil heats up, cook the steak until browned on both sides.

- Whisk the garlic, soy sauce, ginger, beef stock, maple syrup, chilli flakes, Worcestershire sauce and 1 tbsp. cornflour until combined. Add this sauce to the pan and cook for 2-3 minutes.

- Garnish with sliced chilli.

- Serve with rice or a salad.

Salmon with Lemon Butter Sauce

Super simple! A tasty meal any night of the week, and
on your plate in less than 30 minutes.

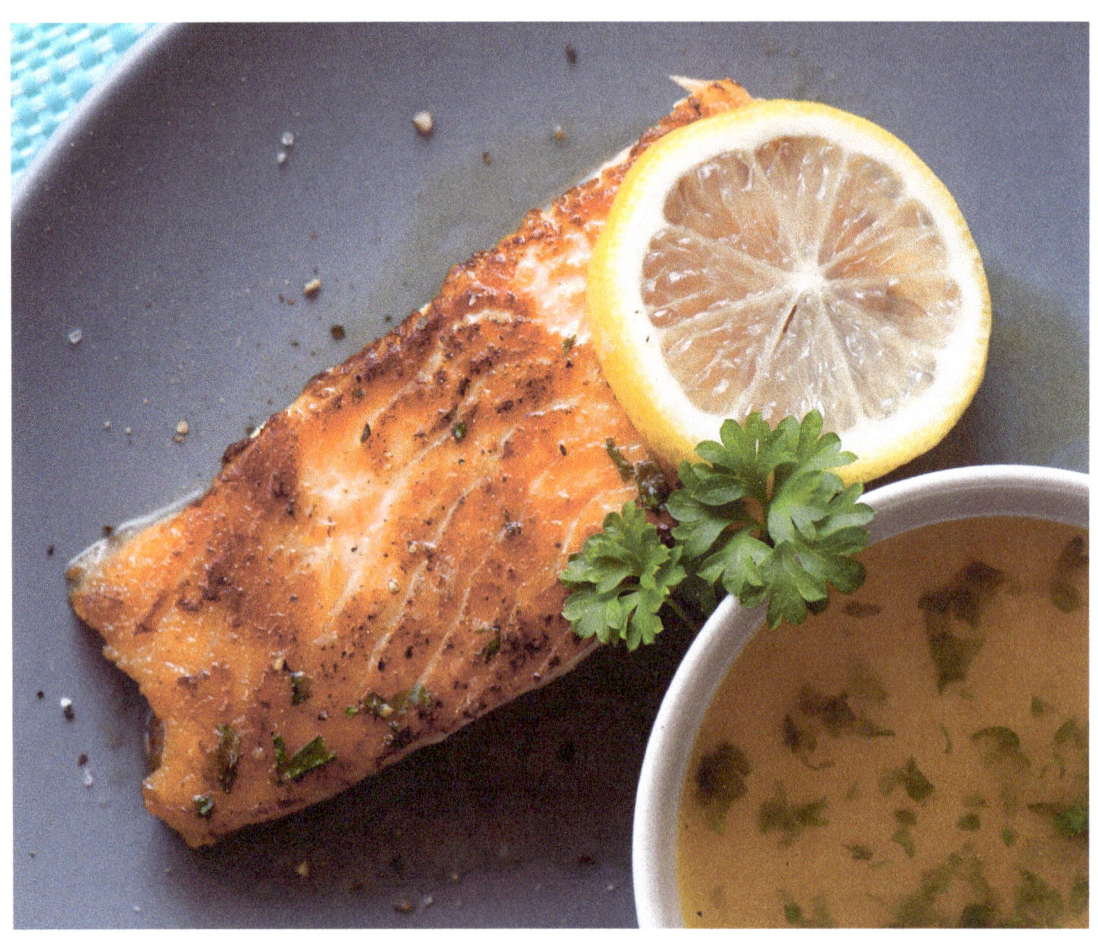

Prep Time: 5 mins | Total Time: 25 mins | Serves: 4

WHAT YOU'LL NEED:

4 salmon fillets	2 tbsp. fresh parsley (chopped)
2 garlic cloves (minced)	¼ cup chicken stock
4 tsp. unsalted butter	Juice of 1 lemon
½ tsp. honey	Lemon slices, to garnish
2 tsp. olive oil	Salt and black pepper, to taste

WHAT TO DO:

- To make the lemon butter sauce: Place a medium pan over medium heat. Add 1 tsp. of butter and allow to melt. Add the garlic and sauté for 1-2 minutes and then pour the chicken stock along with the lemon juice. Allow the sauce to simmer for a few minutes, until reduced. Next, stir in the honey and whisk until combined. Set aside.

- Take paper towels and dab on both sides of the salmon fillets. Season with salt and pepper.

- Heat olive oil in a non-stick pan over medium-high heat and cook the salmon for 4-5 minutes on each side (depending on the thickness of the pieces).

- Place the salmon fillets on a serving plate and drizzle the lemon butter sauce on top. Garnish with lemon slices and serve.

- Serve with rice or salad.

Chilli Beef and Bean Lettuce Wraps

A Mexican style favourite that is nice and light.
A tasty lunch, dinner or snack.

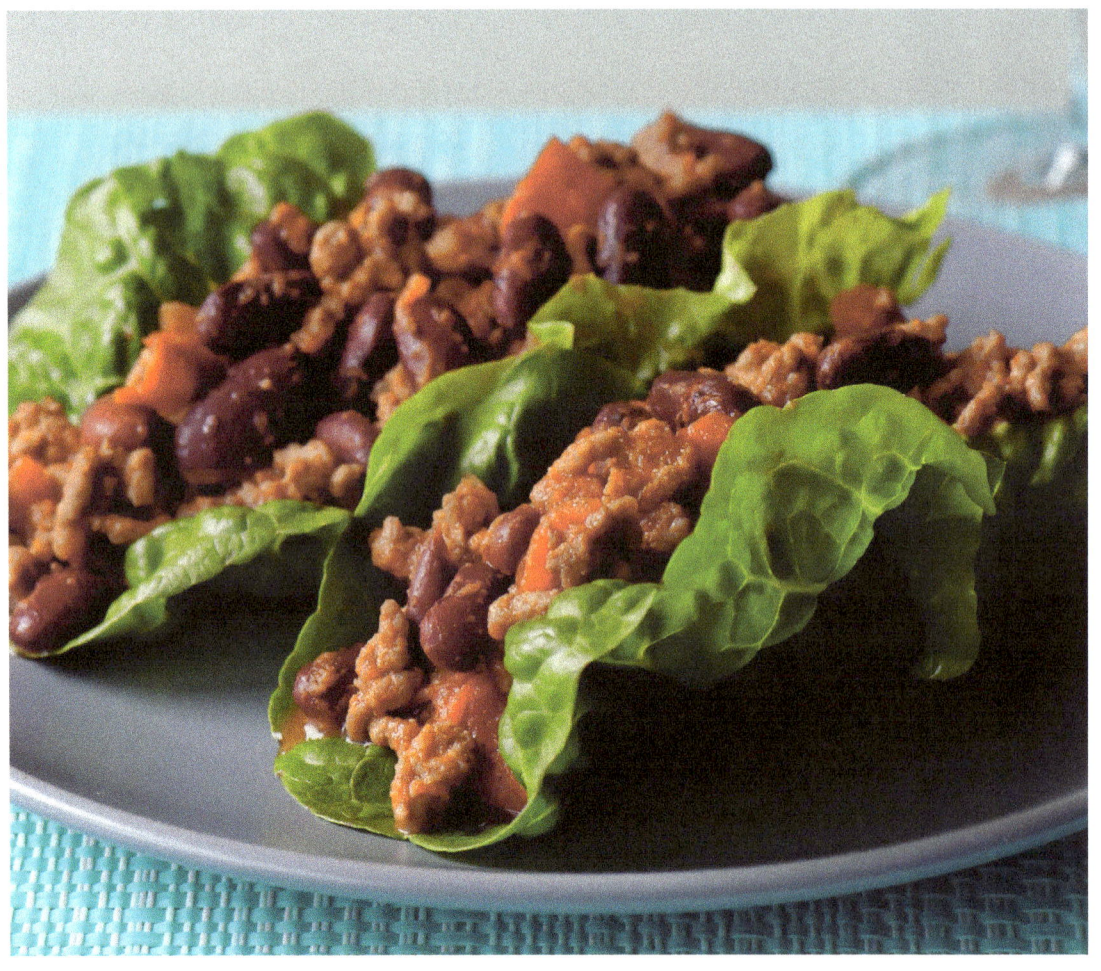

Prep Time: 5 mins | Total Time: 30 mins | Serves: 4

WHAT YOU'LL NEED:

500g lean beef mince

½ red onion (diced)

1 can red kidney beans (rinsed)

1 can diced tomatoes

1 cos lettuce

2 tbsp. tomato paste

½ tsp. chilli powder

¼ tsp. cumin

1 tsp. paprika

1 tsp. garlic powder

Pinch of salt.

WHAT TO DO:

- In a large pan, heat the oil. Add the onion and cook until browned.

- Add the mince, and cook until browned.

- Add in the canned tomatoes, tomato paste, and kidney beans.

- Add the chilli powder, cumin, paprika, garlic powder and salt.

- Allow to simmer until liquid has reduced. Taste and add more chilli powder if desired.

- Serve in lettuce leaves. Wrap and enjoy.

- (Optional - add some sour cream on top.)

SIMPLE SALADS

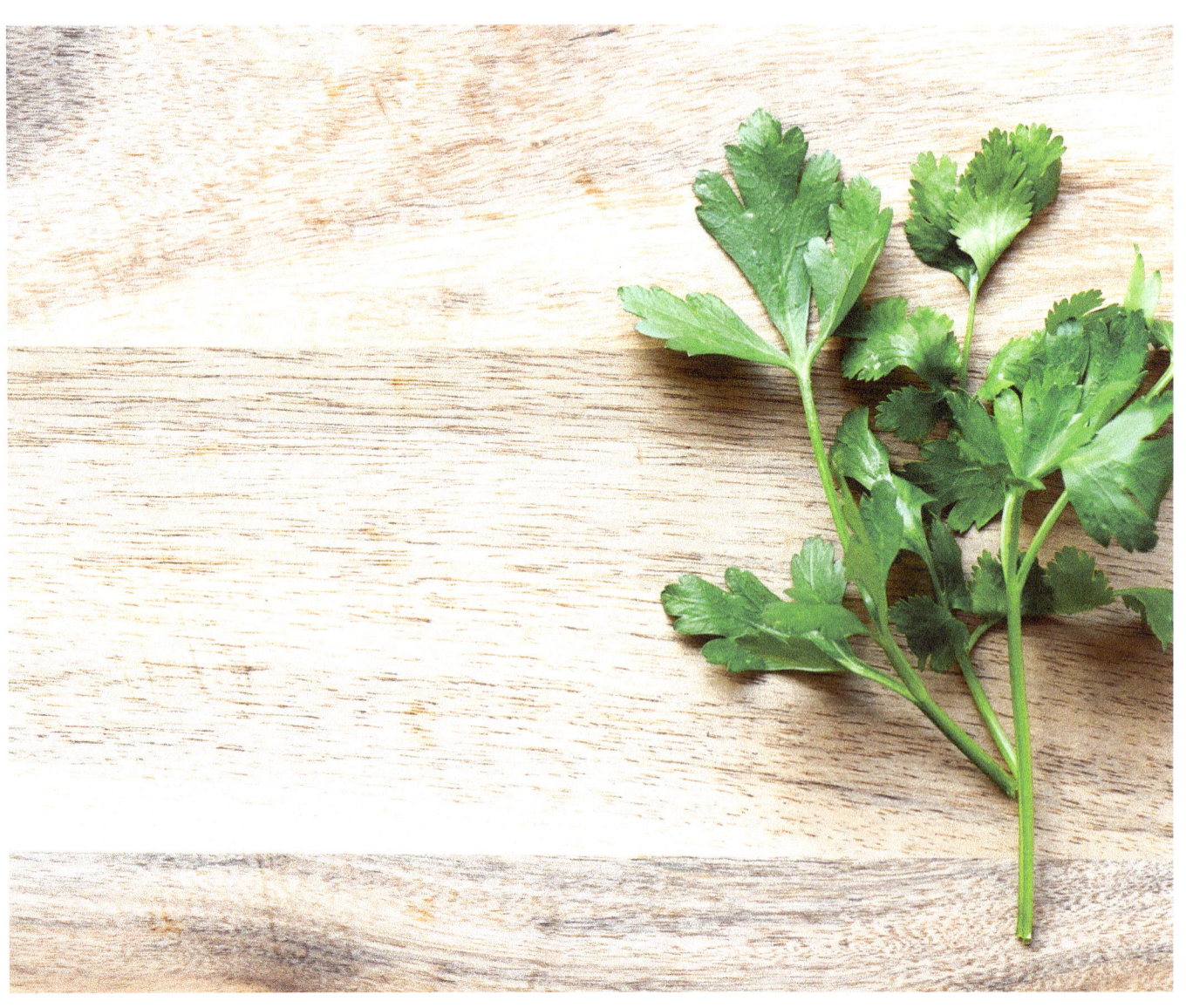

1.   BBQ Chicken Salad

2.   Asian Quinoa and Peanut Salad

3.   Roasted Pumpkin and Mushroom Salad

4.   Asian Tuna and Cucumber Salad

5.   Broccoli Salad

6.   Veggie Salad with Sesame Dressing

7.   Cucumber with Sesame Chicken

8.   Avocado, Chicken and Strawberry Salad

9.   Snow Pea and Quinoa Salad

10.   Classic Chicken Salad

11.   Healthy Tuna Salad

12.   Red Kidney Bean and Avocado Salad

13.   Colourful Kale Salad

14.   Roasted Sweet Potato Salad

BBQ Chicken Salad

This salad looks like a party on a plate!
The bold flavours of the chicken add a very nice touch to
the entire dish.

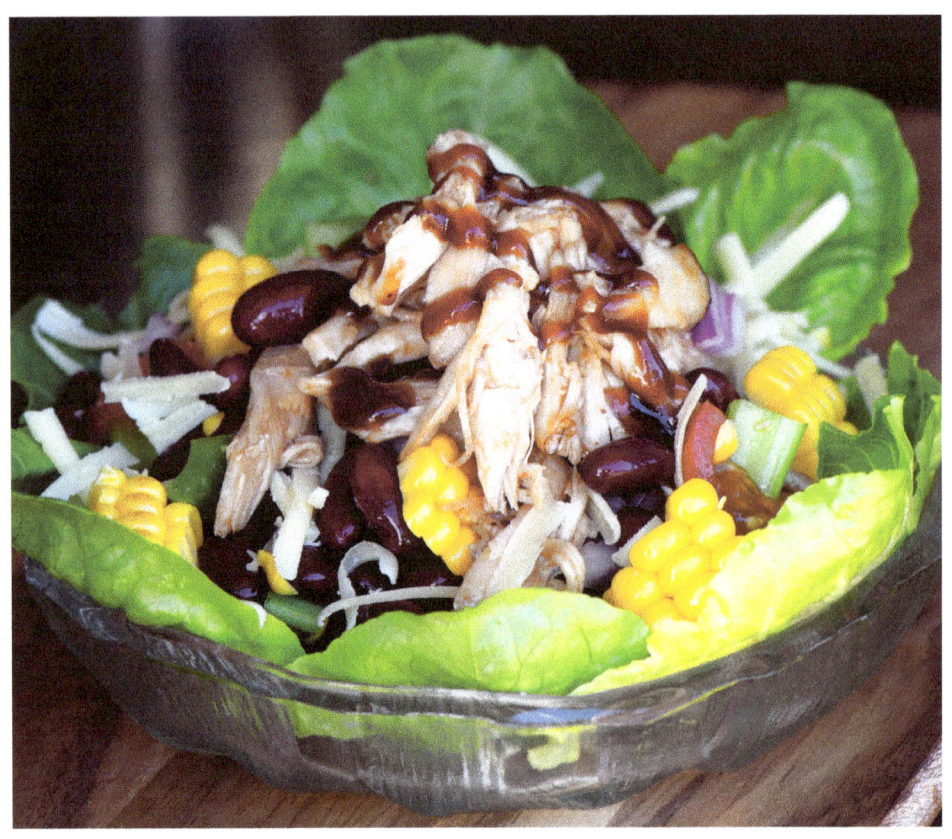

Prep Time: 5 mins | Total Time: 35 mins | Serves: 2-3

WHAT YOU'LL NEED:

2 chicken breasts	1 cup red kidney beans
2 ears sweet corn	½ cup cheddar cheese (grated)
2 chopped Cos lettuce	½ small red onion (diced)
2 tomatoes (diced)	I stick celery (diced)
⅓ cup BBQ sauce	

WHAT TO DO:

- Spray a non-stick pan with cooking spray and place over medium-high heat. Coat the chicken breasts with BBQ sauce. Place chicken into the pan and cook for 5 minutes. Turn over and cook for 5 more minutes. Turn the heat down to low and cook chicken for 20 minutes, turning twice.

- Grill or steam corn until cooked.

- Let the chicken cool down and then shred. Slice the corn kernels off the cob and set both aside.

- Take a large bowl and add the lettuce, tomatoes, red onion, chicken, kidney beans, corn, and cheese.

- Drizzle BBQ sauce over the top.

Asian Quinoa and Peanut Salad

A Thai salad made with healthy and tasty ingredients that make the perfect lunch idea.

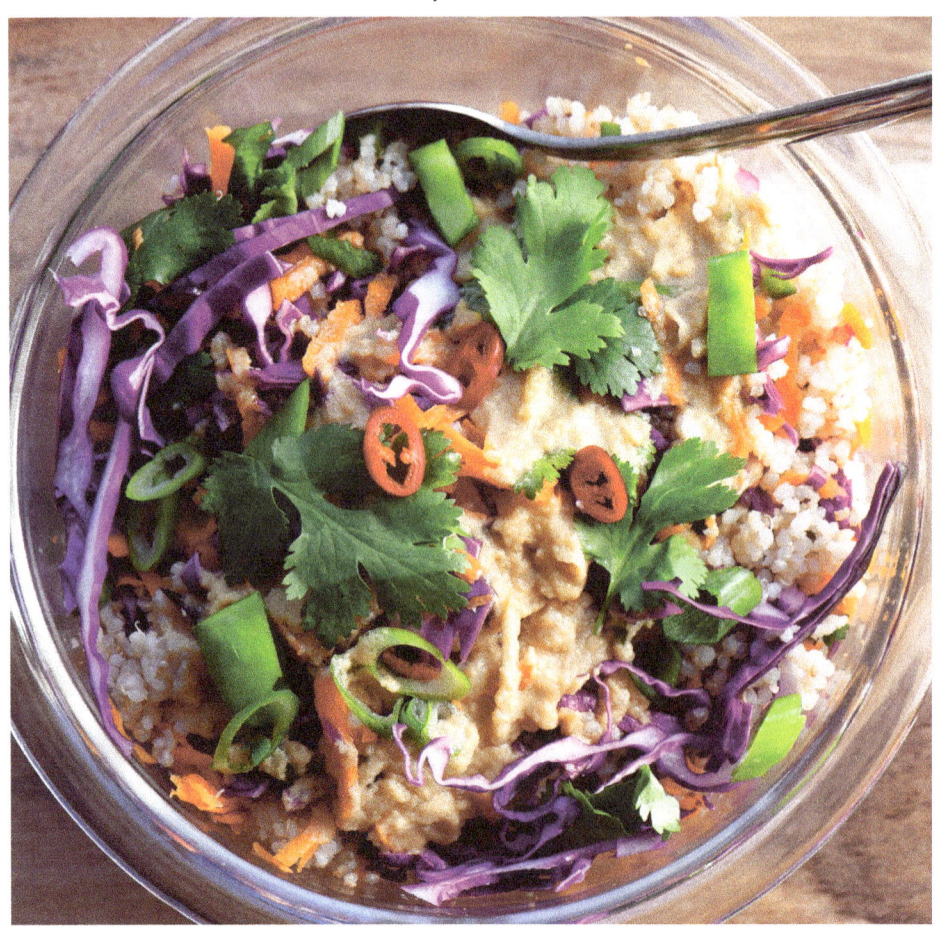

Prep Time: 10 mins | Total Time: 25 mins | Serves: 4

WHAT YOU'LL NEED:

1 cup carrot (grated)

¾ cup uncooked quinoa

1 ½ cups water

½ cup coriander (chopped)

2 cups purple cabbage (shredded)

¼ cup spring onion (sliced)

1 cup snow peas (thinly sliced)

¼ cup roasted peanuts (chopped, for garnish)

FOR THE PEANUT SAUCE:

1 tsp. sesame oil

3 tbsp. soy sauce

1 tbsp. honey

Juice of ½ lime

1 tbsp. rice wine vinegar

½ a chilli sliced

¼ cup peanut butter

1 tsp. grated fresh ginger

WHAT TO DO:

- Rinse the quinoa and add it to a medium-size pot with 1 ½ cup water. Once the mixture comes to a gentle boil, turn the heat down and let it simmer until all water has been absorbed. Take the quinoa off the heat, cover the pot and let it rest for 5 minutes. Afterwards, fluff it with a fork.

- While the quinoa is cooking, make the peanut sauce by whisking the soy sauce and peanut butter together. Add remaining ingredients and whisk again. Add water if the mixture feels too thick.

- In a large bowl, combine the quinoa, snow peas, spring onion, shredded cabbage, coriander and carrot. Pour the peanut sauce over the top

Roasted Pumpkin and Mushroom Salad

Roasted butternut with some sautéed mushrooms makes a really healthy and filling salad.

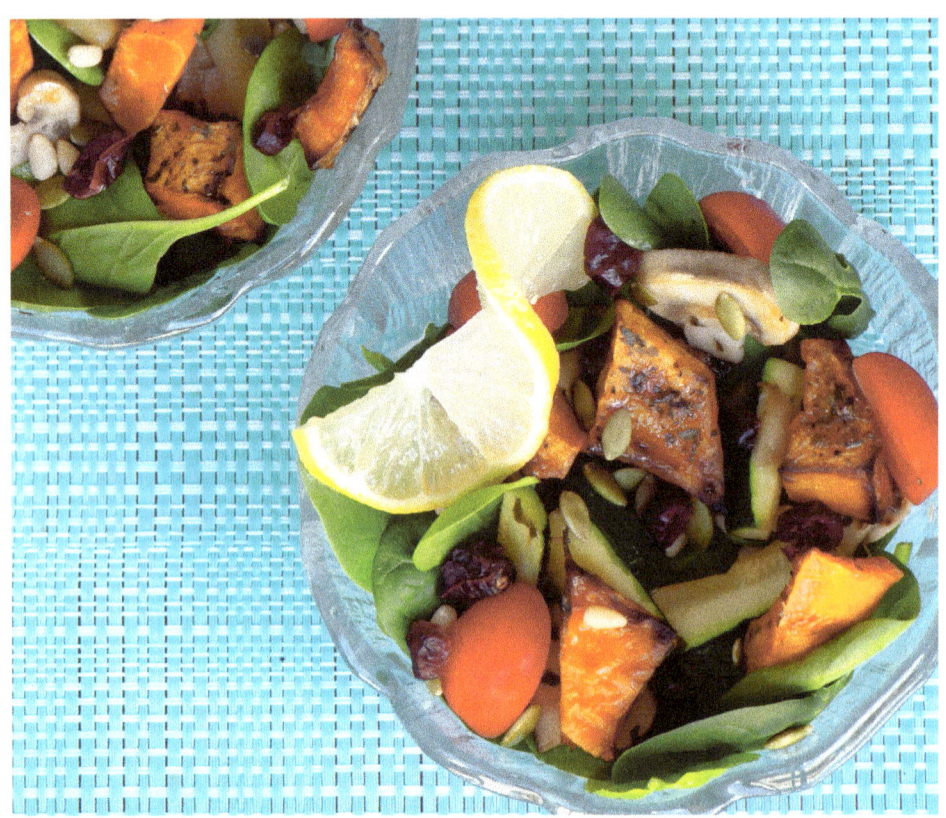

Prep Time: 10 mins | Total Time: 40 mins | Serves: 4

WHAT YOU'LL NEED:

2 cups of baby spinach

1 butternut pumpkin

2 small zucchinis

Dash of olive oil for cooking

¼ cup of mixed pine nuts and pumpkin seeds

½ cup of dried cranberries

1 punnet of cherry tomatoes (halved)

1 cup of mushrooms

4 tsp. dried herbs (any type)

Flaxseed oil (for dressing)

Lime or lemon juice to taste

Dash of olive oil for cooking

WHAT TO DO:

- Preheat oven to 200 degrees.
  Chop the pumpkin into pieces. Place on an oven tray lined with baking paper. Lightly spray with cooking spray, coat with dried herbs. Bake until pumpkin is cooked and set aside to cool.

- Around 10 minutes before the pumpkin is done cooking, add the mushrooms and zucchini to the pan along with some olive oil, and mixed herbs.

- Right before the veggies are done roasting, put the pine nuts and pumpkin seeds on a tray to roast.

- Place a handful of spinach onto each plate. Divide roasted veggies between the plates. Top off with the tomatoes and cranberries. Drizzle the flaxseed oil on top and squeeze on the lemon juice to taste.

Asian Tuna and Cucumber Salad

Quick, easy and healthy salad for lunch.

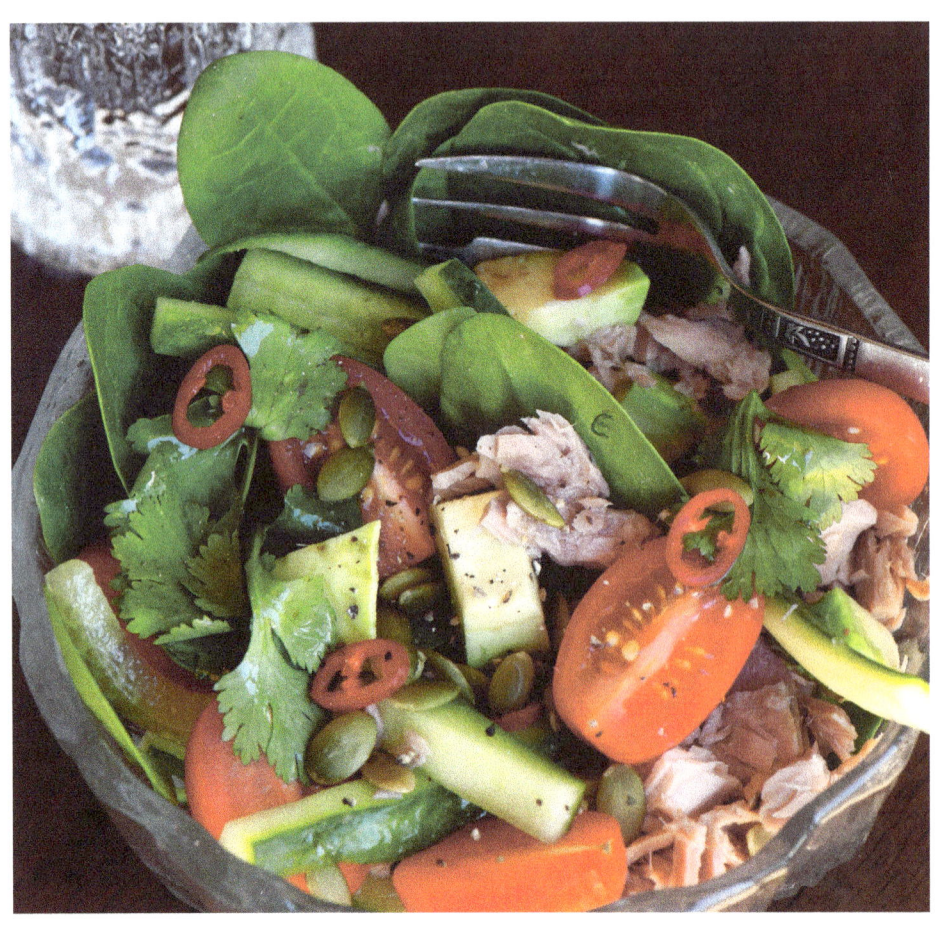

Prep Time: 10 mins | Total Time: 10 mins | Serves: 2

WHAT YOU'LL NEED:

1 cup of baby spinach

2 cucumbers

½ - 1 whole avocado
(diced or sliced)

180g tuna (no salt added)

2 tsp. sesame oil

Lime juice to taste

1 tsp. minced garlic

1 tsp. sliced chilli

2 tbsp. coriander (chopped)

2 tsp. rice wine vinegar

Black pepper, to taste

Sunflower seeds (optional)

WHAT TO DO:

- Slice the cucumbers into thin strips. Pat the cucumber dry to get rid of any excess moisture.

- Put the cucumber into a bowl and add in the rice vinegar and 1 tsp. of sesame oil.

- In another small bowl, add the tuna, garlic, coriander, vinegar, 1 tsp. of sesame oil and pepper. Mix together well.

- Place all the ingredients into two salad bowls. Add a splash of lime juice to taste.

- Garnish with sunflower seeds

Broccoli Salad

This salad recipe isn't just healthy, but super delicious too!
It'll become your new favourite; trust me!

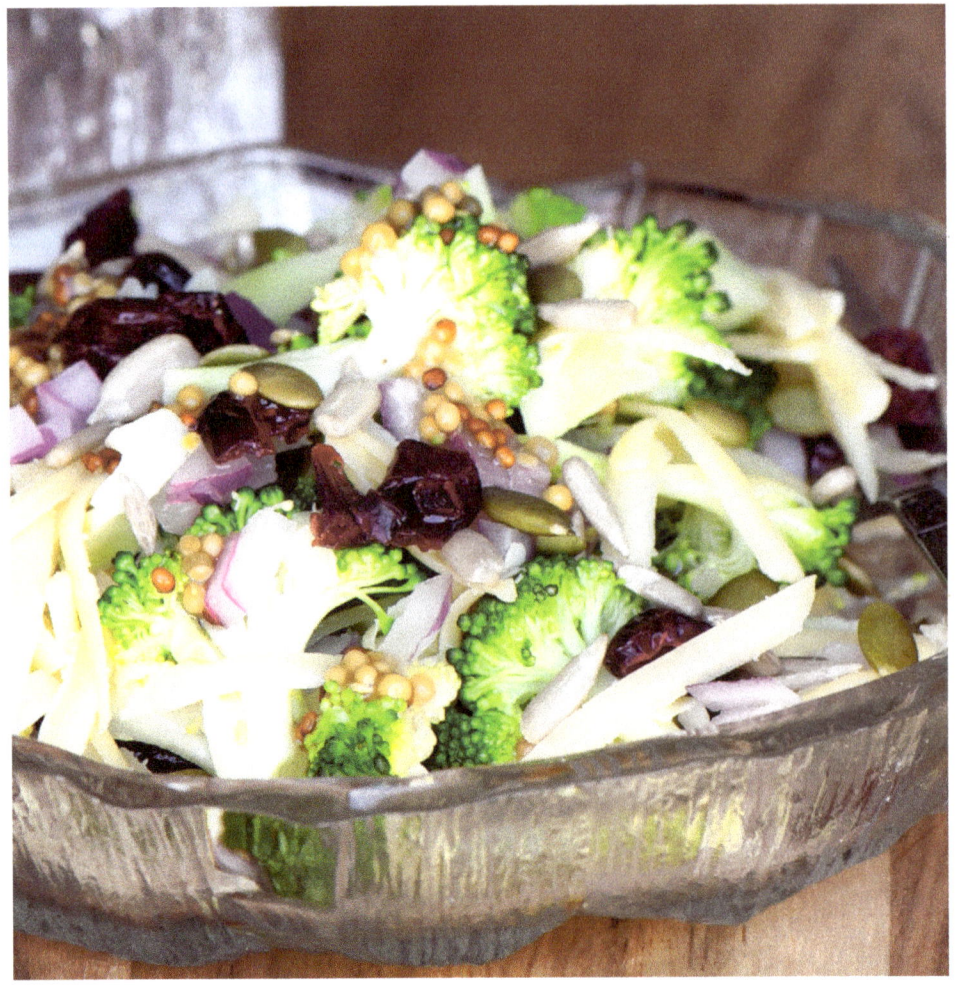

Prep Time: 15 mins | Total Time: 15 mins | Serves: 2

WHAT YOU'LL NEED:

½ cup sunflower seeds

1 broccoli (roughly chopped into small pieces)

½ cup tasty cheese (grated)

⅓ cup dried cranberries (chopped)

½ cup red onion (diced)

FOR THE HONEY MUSTARD DRESSING:

1 tbsp. honey

⅓ cup extra-virgin olive oil

1 medium garlic clove (minced)

2 tbsp. apple cider vinegar

¼ tsp. fine sea salt

1 tbsp. wholegrain mustard

WHAT TO DO:

- Add the sunflower seeds into a pan over medium heat and cook them for 5 minutes while stirring frequently. Once toasted, add them to a large bowl.

- Steam the broccoli for only a minute or two, so it still has crunch.

- Make the honey mustard sauce by combining all ingredients in a small bowl and whisk until well blended.

- Add the onion, cranberries, broccoli and cheese into the same bowl.

- Pour the dressing over the salad and stir until coated.

Veggie Salad with Sesame Dressing

This salad features all the Asian flavours you know and love.

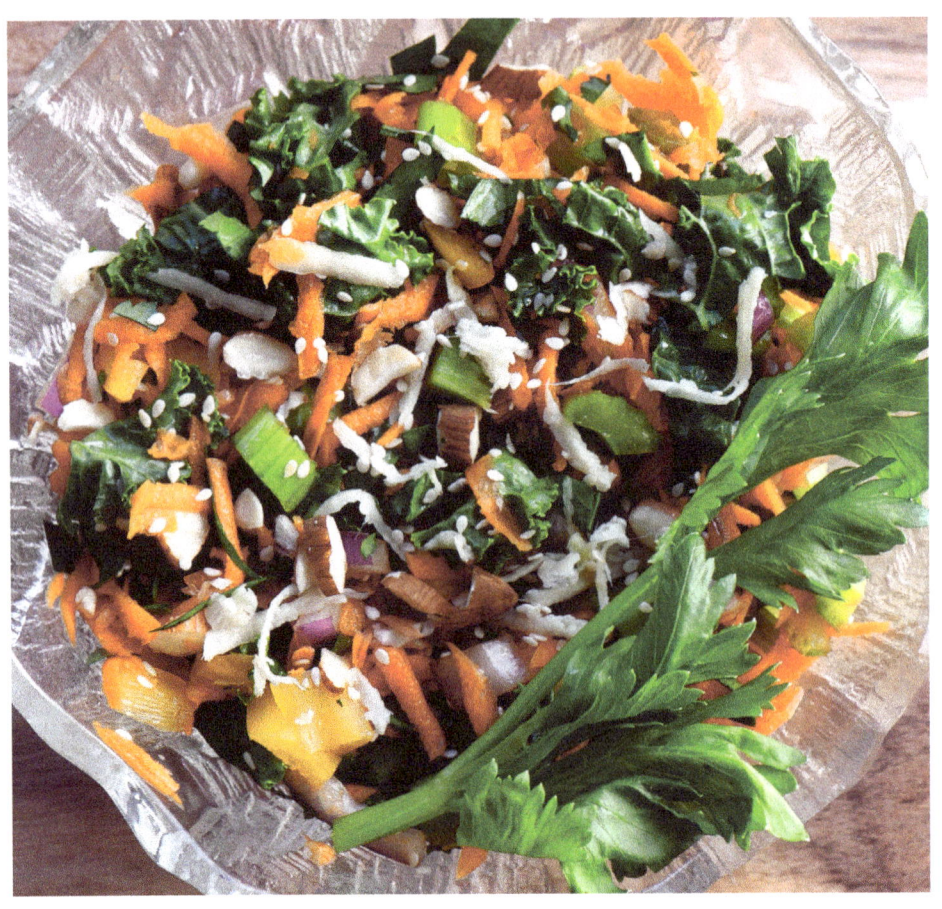

Prep Time: 15 mins | Total Time: 15 mins | Serves: 2-3

WHAT YOU'LL NEED:

2 celery stalks (finely diced)

¼ cup parsley or coriander (chopped)

2 carrots (grated)

2 tbsp. sesame seeds

1 red capsicum (finely diced)

¼ medium red onion (finely diced)

1 leaf of kale (de-stemmed and sliced)

¼ cup roasted almonds or peanuts

FOR THE DRESSING:

1 tsp. grated ginger

2 tbsp. sesame oil

1 tbsp. honey

1 small garlic clove (minced)

1 tbsp. lemon juice

2 tsp. soy sauce

WHAT TO DO:

- Whisk dressing ingredients in a small bowl and set aside.
- Toss salad ingredients together and a large bowl and drizzle dressing over top.
- Toss to coat.

Cucumber with Sesame Chicken

This refreshing salad features Asian flavours and is the best way to use leftover chicken.

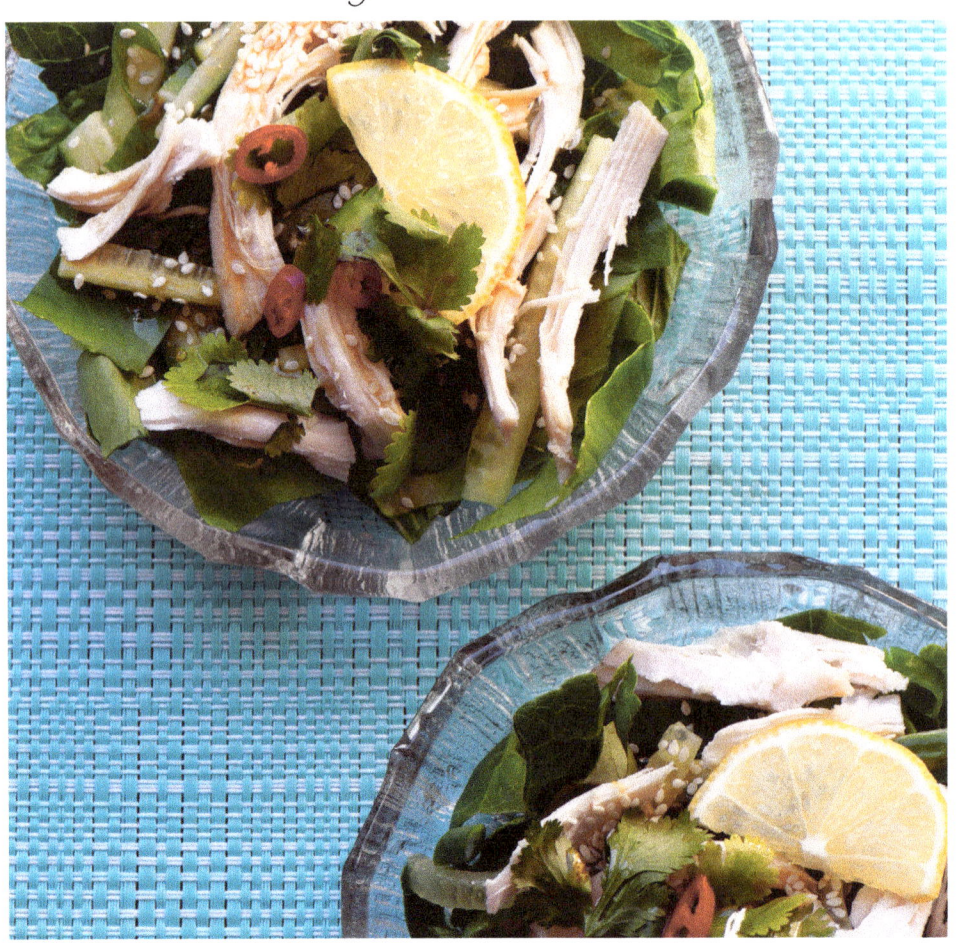

Prep Time: 15 mins | Total Time: 15 mins | Serves: 4

WHAT YOU'LL NEED:

2 cucumbers

2-3 cups of cooked chicken (shredded)

2 tbsp. sesame seeds

3 spring onions (thinly sliced)

1 bunch of bok-choi (shredded)

¼ cup of fresh coriander

1 Cos lettuce (shredded)

1 finely chopped red chilli (to garnish)

FOR THE SESAME DRESSING:

2 tsp. raw honey

5 tbsp. sesame oil

1 tsp. soy sauce

3 tbsp. lemon juice

WHAT TO DO:

- In a dry pan, toast your sesame seeds until fragrant.

- Slice the cucumbers into thin strips. Pat the cucumber dry to get rid of any excess moisture.

- Make the dressing by whisking all the ingredients together.

- In a large bowl, add the bok-choi, lettuce, coriander and spring onion.
  Pour in the dressing and toss to coat.

- Add the shredded chicken and top with toasted sesame seeds.

Avocado, Chicken and Strawberry Salad

A simple balsamic dressing that works as a marinade too! This fresh, healthy and tasty salad will become your go-to.

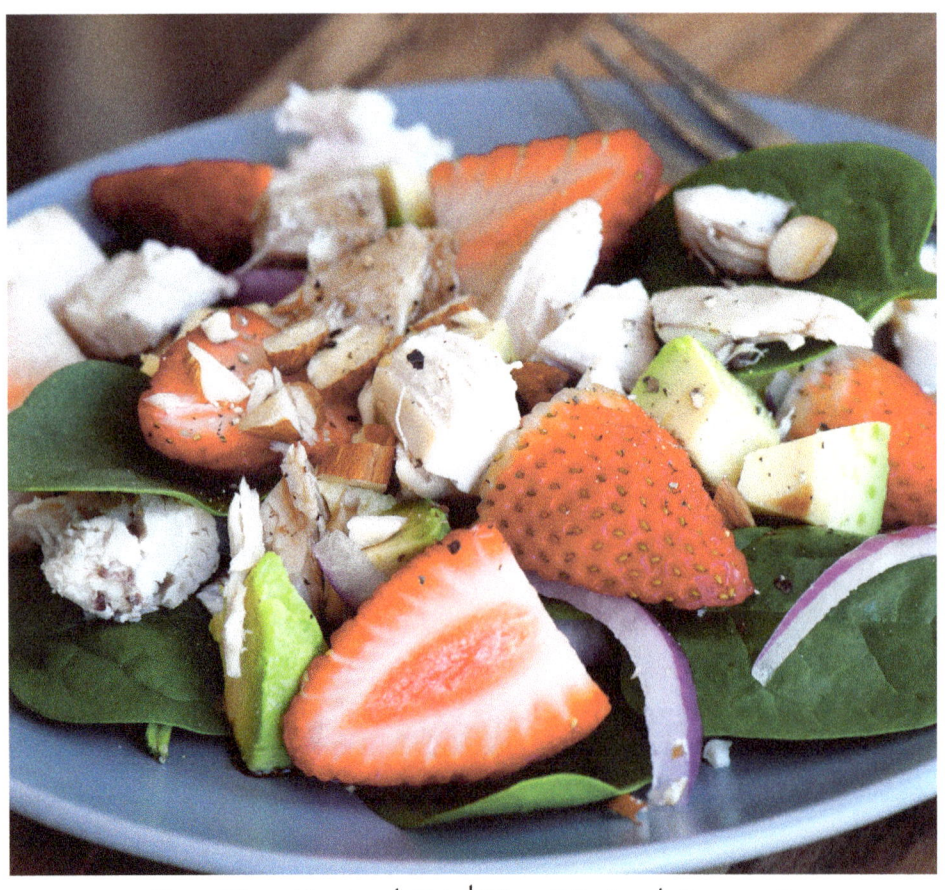

Prep Time: 10 mins | Total Time: 35 mins | Serves: 2

WHAT YOU'LL NEED:

2 chicken breasts

1 avocado (diced)

2 cups baby spinach

½ red onion sliced

1 punnet of strawberries

2 tbsp. sliced almonds

FOR THE MARINADE:

1 tbsp. balsamic vinegar

1 tsp. sugar

½ tsp. ground black pepper

¼ tsp. sea salt

¼ cup extra virgin olive oil

WHAT TO DO:

- Whisk the balsamic vinegar, olive oil, sugar, salt and pepper together in a small bowl.

- Coat the chicken in the dressing.

- Spray a non-stick pan with cooking spray and place over medium-high heat. Coat the chicken breasts with BBQ sauce. Place chicken into the pan and cook for 5 minutes. Turn over and cook for 5 more minutes. Turn the heat down to low and cook chicken for 20 minutes, turning twice.

- Place the red onion, spinach and strawberries in a bowl.

- Drizzle the remaining dressing and add in the sliced chicken and avocado.

- Add sliced almonds on top. Add black pepper to taste

Snow Pea and Quinoa Salad

A colourful salad with snow peas, mushrooms and fresh lemon flavour.

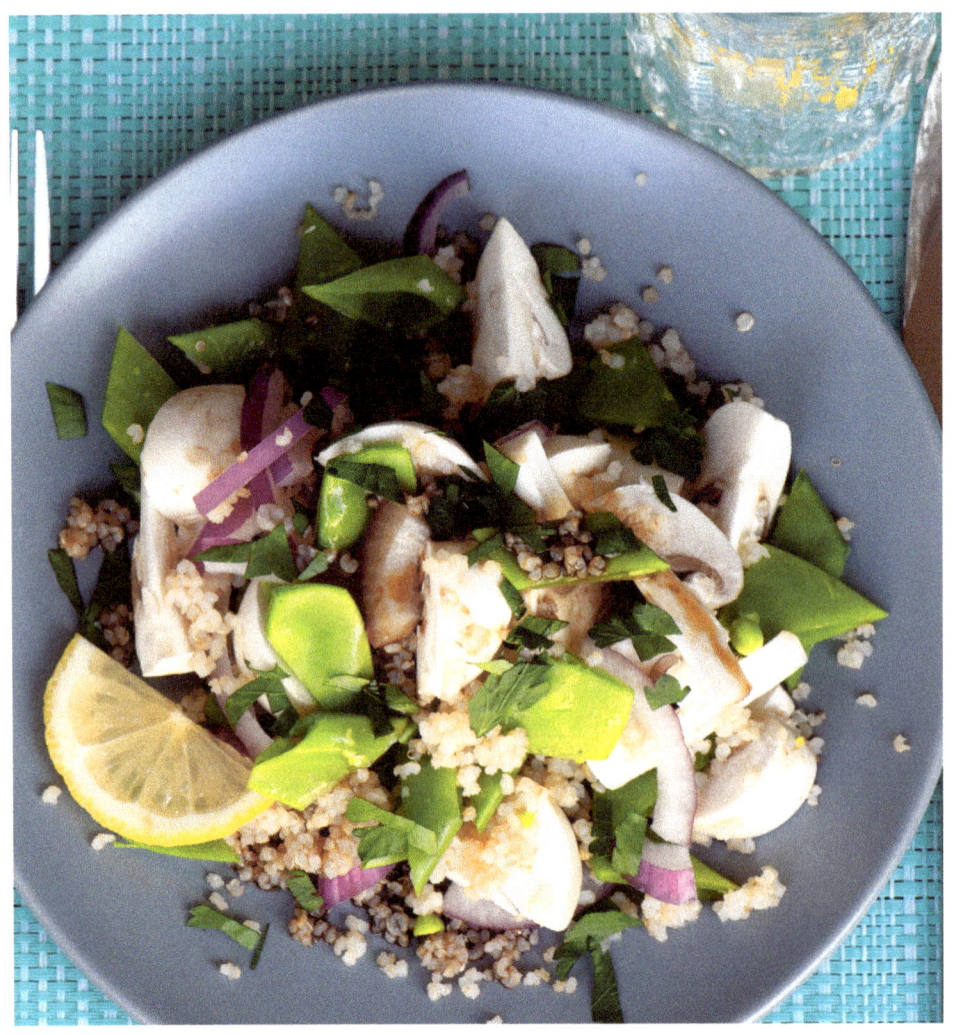

Prep time: 10 mins | Total time: 25 mins | Serves 4

WHAT YOU'LL NEED

¾ cup uncooked quinoa

⅓ cup balsamic vinegar

1½ cups water

1 tbsp. lemon juice

1½ cups button mushrooms
(cut into quarters)

1 tsp. lemon zest
(freshly grated)

2 cups fresh snow peas
(cut diagonally into thirds)

1 tsp. honey

¼ cup fresh parsley
(chopped)

⅓ cup red onion (thinly sliced)

WHAT TO DO:

- Rinse the quinoa and add it to a medium-size pot with 1 ½ cup water. Once the mixture comes to a gentle boil, turn the heat down and let it simmer until all water has been absorbed. Take the quinoa off the heat, cover the pot and let it rest for 5 minutes.
Afterwards, fluff it with a fork.

- In a medium sized bowl, whisk the lemon zest, vinegar, lemon juice and honey together. Add the quinoa and mix through.

- Add peas, mushrooms, parsley and onions and toss.

- Serve.

Classic Chicken Salad

This classic salad becomes so much easier to put together when you top it off with some already cooked BBQ chicken.

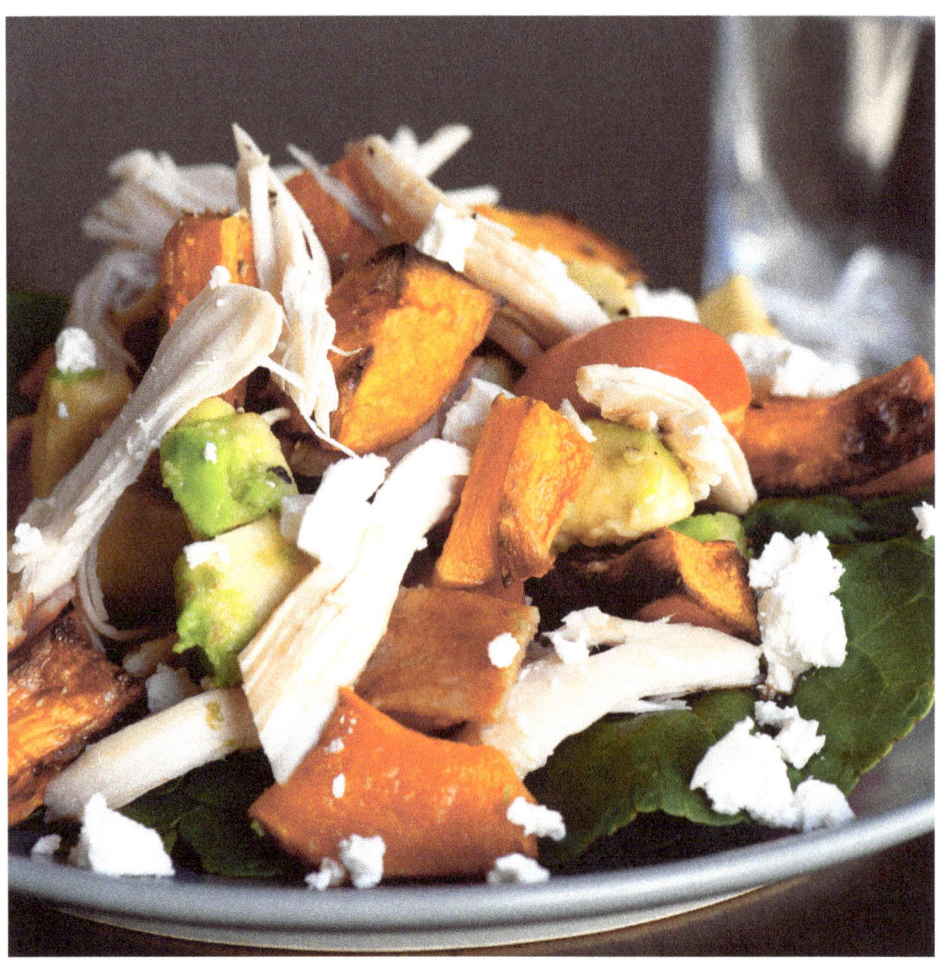

Prep Time: 10 mins | Total Time: 50 mins | Serves: 4

WHAT YOU'LL NEED:

1 avocado (diced)

½ a butternut pumpkin

1 BBQ chicken (or other cooked chicken)

2 tbsp. olive oil (for cooking)

4 large leaves of lettuce (Cos or Iceberg lettuce)

½ a punnet of cherry tomatoes (halved)

4 rashers of bacon

¼ cup crumbled danish feta

Balsamic vinegar to taste.

Flaxseed oil to taste

WHAT TO DO:

- Preheat oven to 200 degrees.
  Chop the pumpkin into pieces. Place on an oven tray lined with baking paper. Lightly spray with cooking spray. Bake until pumpkin is cooked (approximately 45 minutes). Set aside to cool.

- Fry bacon in a pan until cooked. Set aside and slice.

- Shred the BBQ chicken and place in bowl. Add bacon, avocado, danish feta, roasted pumpkin, and tomatoes and toss together.

- Serve the salad on top of each leaf of lettuce.

- Dress with balsamic vinegar and flaxseed oil.

- (Optional - Roasted beetroot is also a nice addition to this salad.)

Healthy Tuna Salad

It's crunchy, it's sweet and it's better than your average salad. Whip it together in 10 minutes and enjoy.

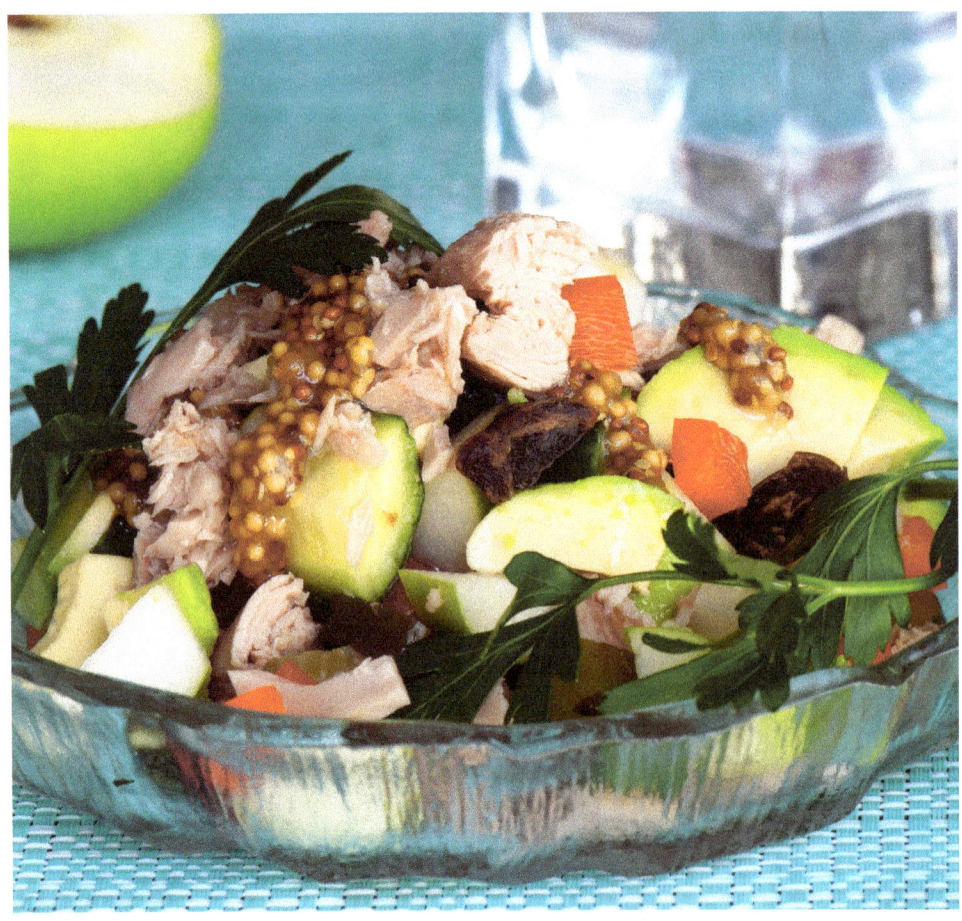

Prep Time: 10 mins | Total Time: 10 mins | Serves: 2

WHAT YOU'LL NEED:

1 cucumber (diced)

180g tuna (no salt added)

2 dates (sliced)

1 apple (diced)

1 red capsicum (diced)

1 avocado (sliced)

1 gherkin (sliced)

FOR THE DRESSING:

2 tbsp. olive oil or flaxseed oil

1 tsp. sea salt

2 tbsp. wholegrain mustard

1 tsp. ground black pepper

½ tsp. paprika

WHAT TO DO:

- Make the dressing by whisking all ingredients together in a small bowl and set aside.

- Drain the tuna and add it to a large bowl. Add the remaining salad ingredients and toss.

- Pour the dressing on top.

Red Kidney Bean and Avocado Salad

A healthy and nutritious salad that serves as a filling meal for everyone.

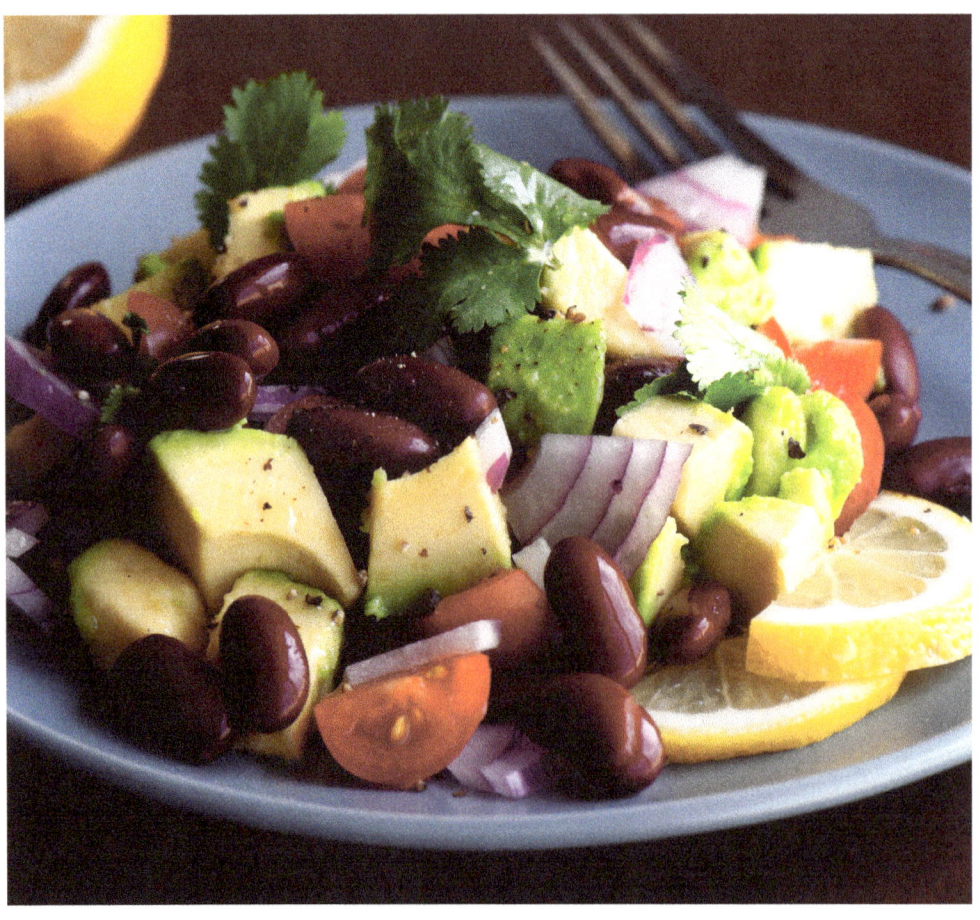

Prep Time: 10 mins | Total Time: 10 mins | Serves: 2

WHAT YOU'LL NEED:

2 tbsp. olive oil or flaxseed oil

1 tomato (chopped)

1 garlic clove
(minced)

½ cup red onion (chopped)

2 avocados (diced)

1 cup red kidney beans
(drained and rinsed)

¼ cup fresh coriander
(chopped)

Juice of 1 lime

Ground black pepper to taste

WHAT TO DO:

- Whisk the lime juice, olive oil, garlic, salt and pepper together in a small bowl.

- Combine the remaining ingredients in a large bowl and drizzle the dressing over the top.

- Toss to coat.

Colourful Kale Salad

This tasty vegan salad features a tangy lemon dressing and sends you on a rollercoaster ride. Also a perfect side dish.

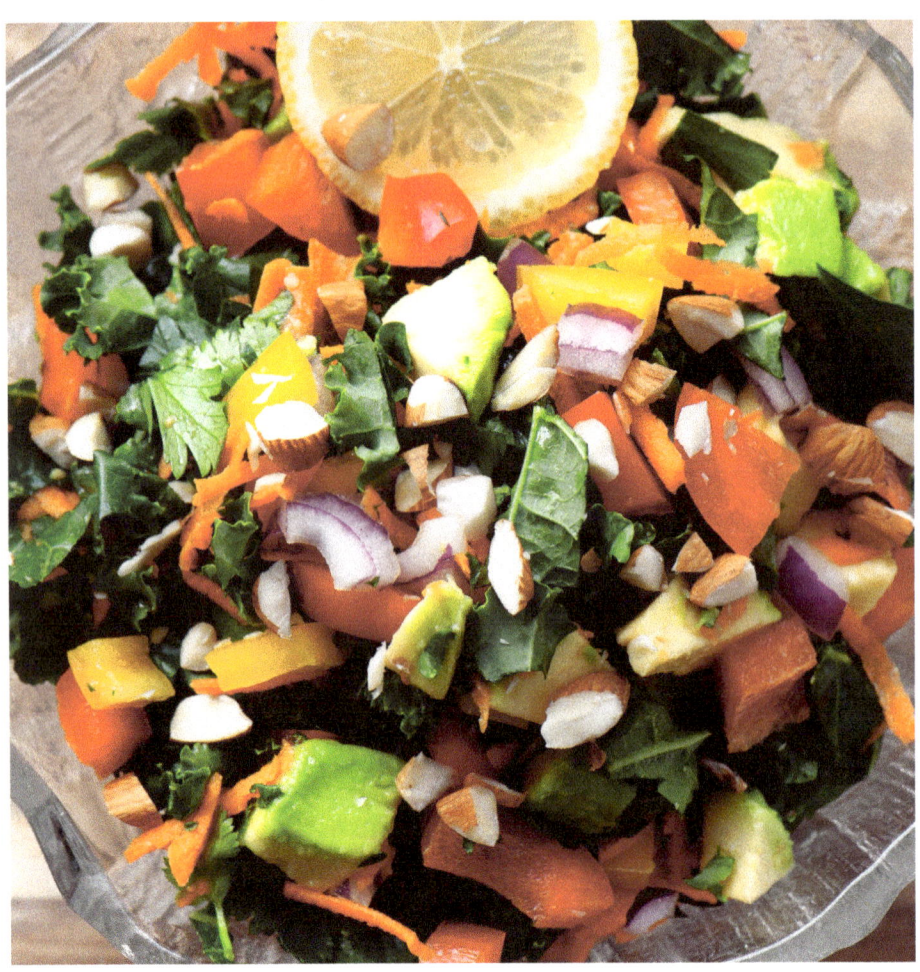

Prep Time: 15 mins | Total Time: 15 mins | Serves: 2-3

WHAT YOU'LL NEED:

1 cup grated carrots

2 capsicum (diced)
(red and yellow for colour)

¼ cup roasted almonds

2 bunches kale
(de-stemmed and finely
chopped)

½ cup coriander (chopped)

½ small red onion (diced)

1 avocado (diced)

⅓ cup parsley (chopped)

FOR THE VINAIGRETTE:

2 tsp. olive oil

½ tsp. sugar

Juice of 1 lemon

2 garlic cloves (minced)

Black pepper, to taste

WHAT TO DO:

- Make the dressing by whisking all ingredients together in a small bowl.

- For the salad, combine all ingredients (except avocado and almonds) together.
  Add the dressing and mix in well.

- Top with avocado and almonds.

Roasted Sweet Potato Salad

This salad features ingredients that make the perfect match when put together. Drizzle the honey lemon dressing on top and you have a delicious salad ready.

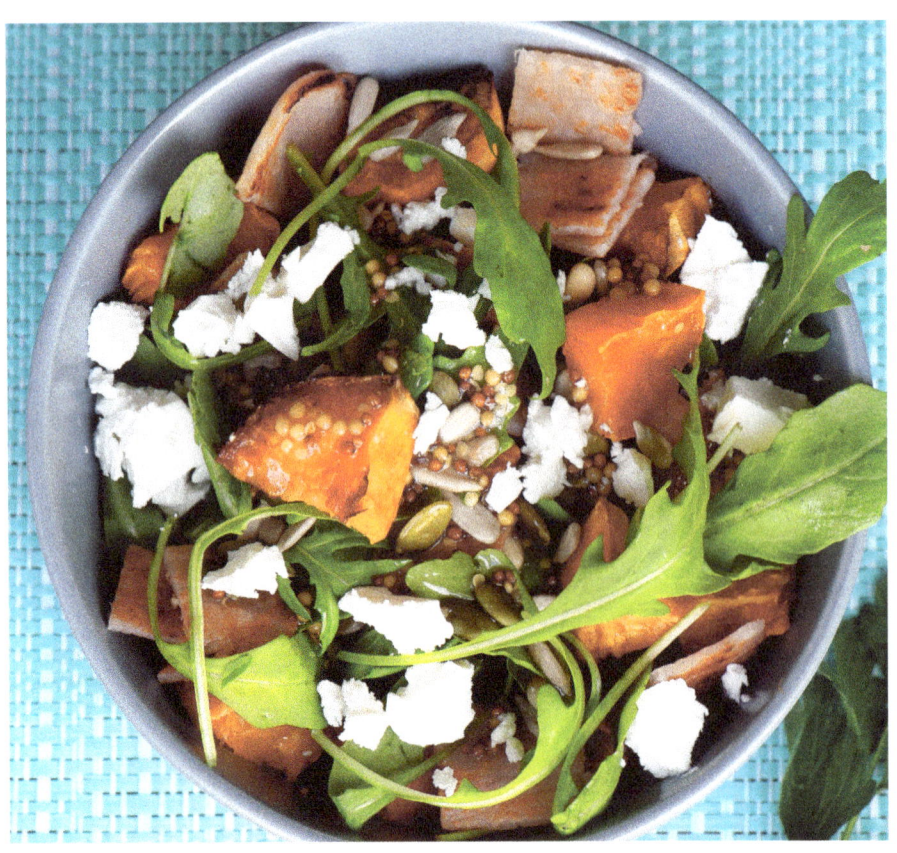

Prep Time: 15 mins | Total Time: 45 mins | Serves: 4

WHAT YOU'LL NEED:

3 cups sweet potato

100g rocket (1 bag)

1 cup danish feta

100g bacon (chopped)

Sprinkle of Sunflower seeds

Sprinkle of Pine nuts

FOR THE HONEY LEMON DRESSING:

2 tbsp. extra virgin olive oil

1 tbsp. honey

½ tsp. wholegrain mustard

2 tbsp. lemon juice

WHAT TO DO:

- Preheat oven to 200 degrees.
  Peel and slice the sweet potato into pieces. Place on an oven tray lined with baking paper. Lightly spray with cooking spray. Bake until sweet potato is cooked (approximately 30 minutes). Set aside to cool.

- Add all ingredients of the dressing together in a small bowl and combine well.

- Fry bacon in a pan until cooked. Set aside and slice.

- Place everything into a bowl (except bacon, cheese, nuts and seeds). Drizzle the dressing in and toss to coat.

- Add the bacon, seeds, nuts and cheese on top and serve.

SIMPLE SMOOTHIES

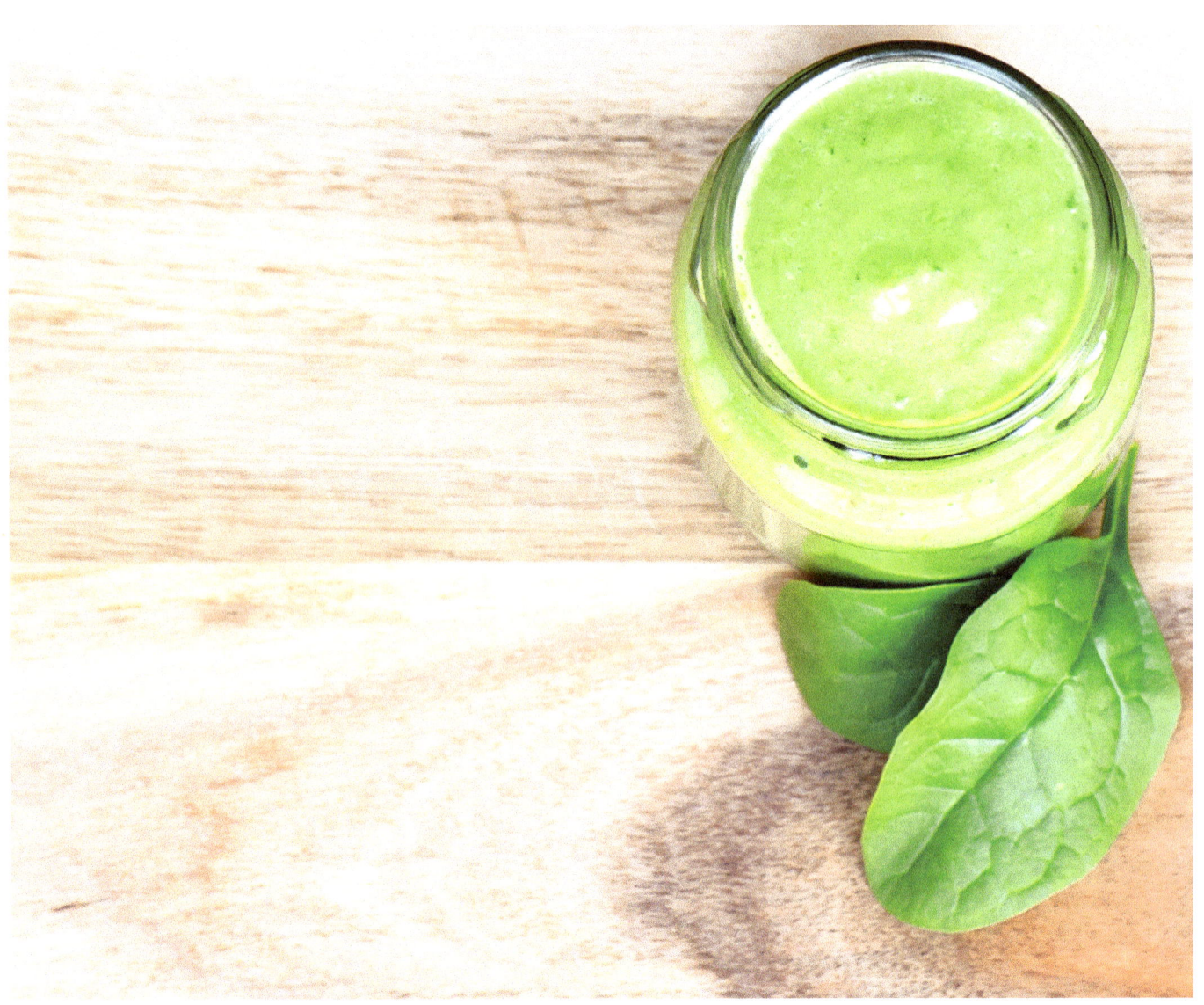

1. Strawberry Orange Smoothie

2. Blueberry Smoothie

3. Refreshing Citrus Smoothie

4. Avocado and Spinach Smoothie

5. Kiwi Avocado Smoothie

6. Green Protein Smoothie

7. Banana Honey Smoothie

8. Raspberry Smoothie

9. Healthy Spinach Smoothie

10. Just Peachy Smoothie

11. Cacao Heaven Smoothie

12. Beetroot Cinnamon Smoothie

13. Orange Mango Smoothie

14. Carrot and Mango Smoothie

15. Blackberry Cheesecake Smoothie

Smoothies are a great way to help reach the daily recommended intake of fruits and vegetables into your day. Provide your body with the nutrition it needs to thrive.

Maca powder, Acai powder, greens powder, hemp seeds, chia seeds and protein powders can be added to any smoothies to give your body the nutrient and fibre boost it needs.

A note on protein powders - use whatever works for you! There are so many out there, milk based, plant based, lactose free, and all at a differing cost. The best guide is to look for one that is natural, high in protein and low in added sugars.

Any of these smoothies can be turned into smoothie bowls. Thicken the mix by using frozen fruit or more ice cubes. Pour into a bowl, place nuts, fruit, seeds on top, and enjoy with a spoon.

Strawberry Orange Smoothie

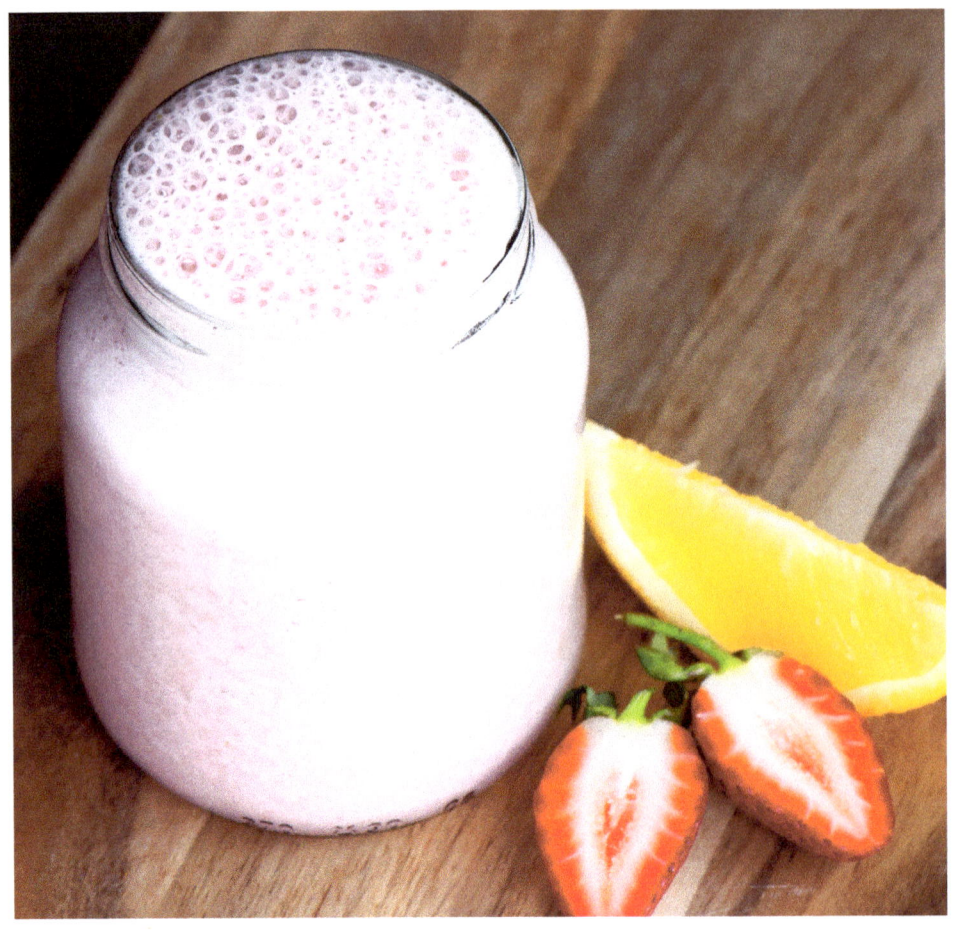

Prep time: 5 mins | Serves 1

You can't go wrong with the simple sweet flavours of strawberries and orange.

WHAT YOU'LL NEED:

1 tsp. Acai powder

¼ cup of strawberries

½ an orange

1 small carrot

1 small banana

½ scoop of protein powder

½ cup water

6-8 ice cubes

WHAT TO DO:

- De-stem strawberries, peel orange and remove seeds and peel the banana.

- Simply place all ingredients in a blender and blend until smooth.

Acai berries are rich in antioxidants and vitamin C.
The Acai powder has a slightly bitter taste that is balanced out with the sweetness of the other fruits.

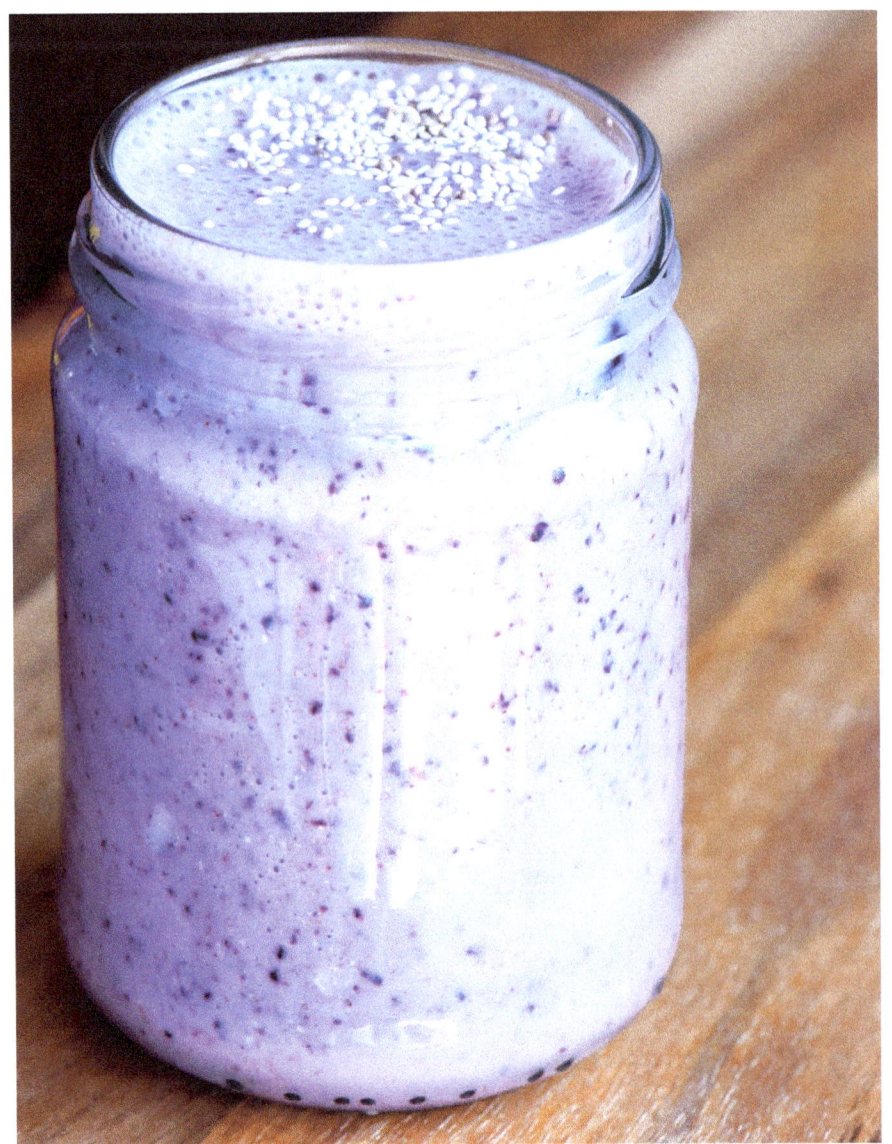

Prep time: 5 mins | Serves 1

Blueberry Smoothie

WHAT YOU'LL NEED:

½ cup of blueberries

½ cup almond milk

1 tsp. of cinnamon

¼ cup of chia seeds

½ cup coconut milk

WHAT TO DO:

• Simply place all ingredients in a blender and blend until smooth.

If fresh blueberries are not in season, substitute with frozen ones.

Refreshing Citrus Smoothie

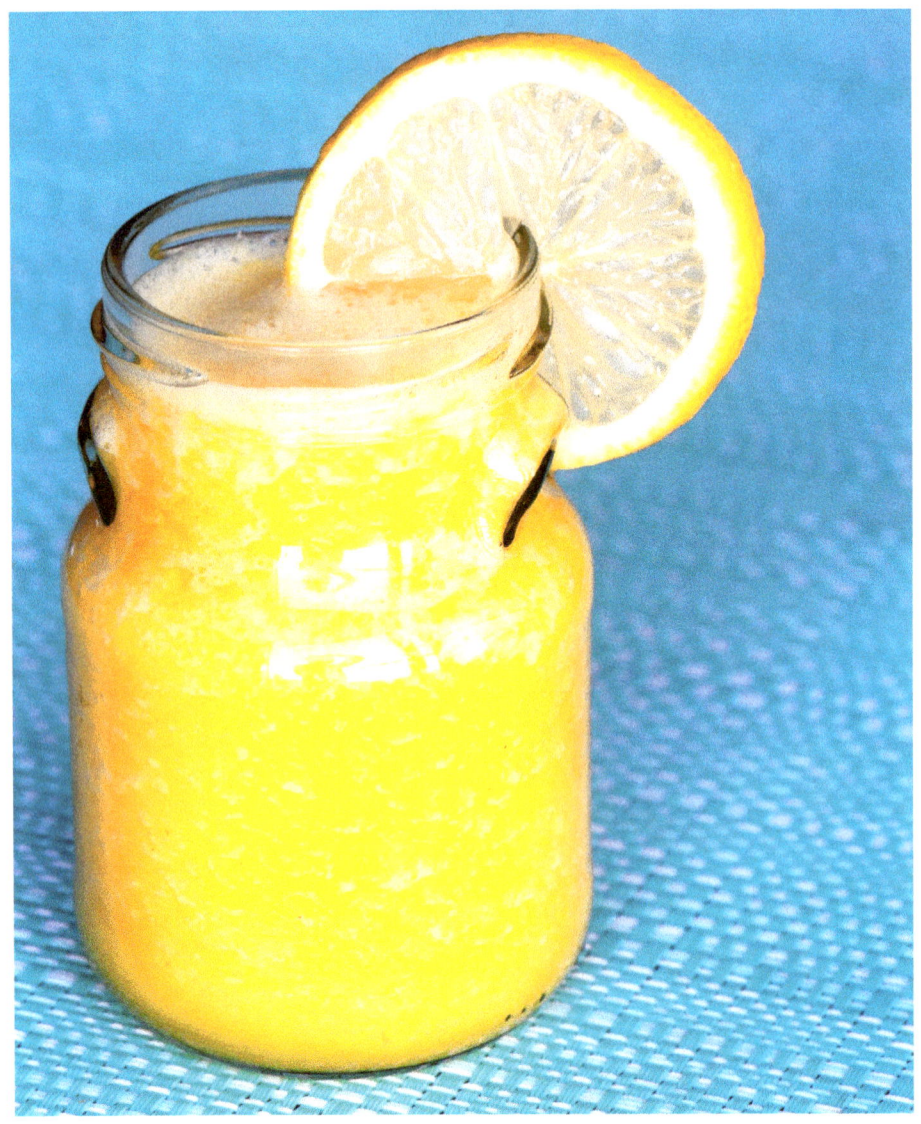

Prep time: 5 mins | Serves 1

Citrus with a bite! A refreshing bitter flavour to make your taste buds tingle.

WHAT YOU'LL NEED:

½ a lemon	½ cup of water
¼ a grapefruit	Small slice of ginger
1 orange	¼ tsp. of Maca powder
1 tbsp. honey	Sprinkle of turmeric

WHAT TO DO:

- Peel citrus and remove seeds.

- Simply place all ingredients in a blender and blend until smooth.

Maca powder contains essential amino acids, calcium, magnesium, and potassium. It also contains protein and fibre. It has an earthy taste, which to a new user can be a little overwhelming, use sparingly for the first time.

Avocado and Spinach Smoothie

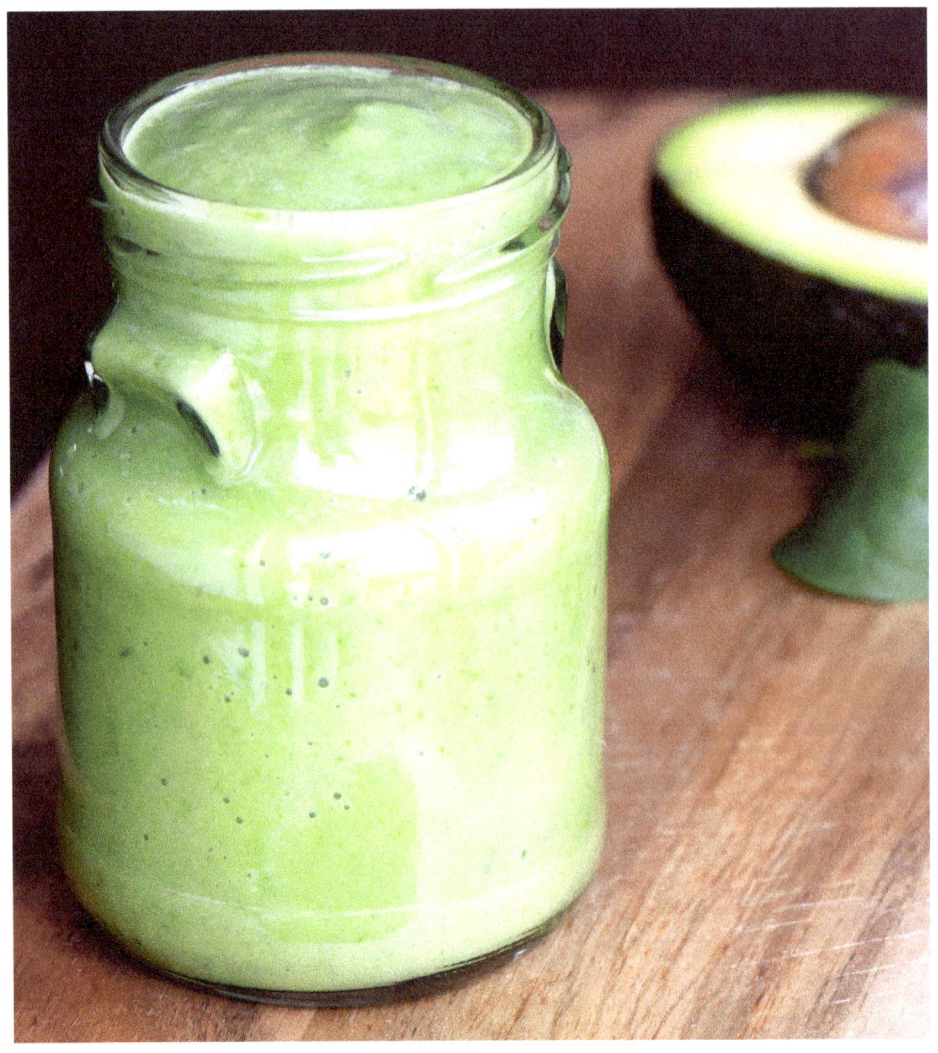

Prep time: 5 mins | Serves 1

An everyday go to. A beautiful creamy smoothie packed with nutrients and essential oils your body will love you for.

WHAT YOU'LL NEED:

2 cups of baby spinach

½ an avocado

1 apple

1 cup of water

6-8 ice cubes

WHAT TO DO:

- Peel and remove seed from avocado. Remove core from apple.

- Simply place all ingredients in a blender and blend until smooth.

Kiwi Avocado Smoothie

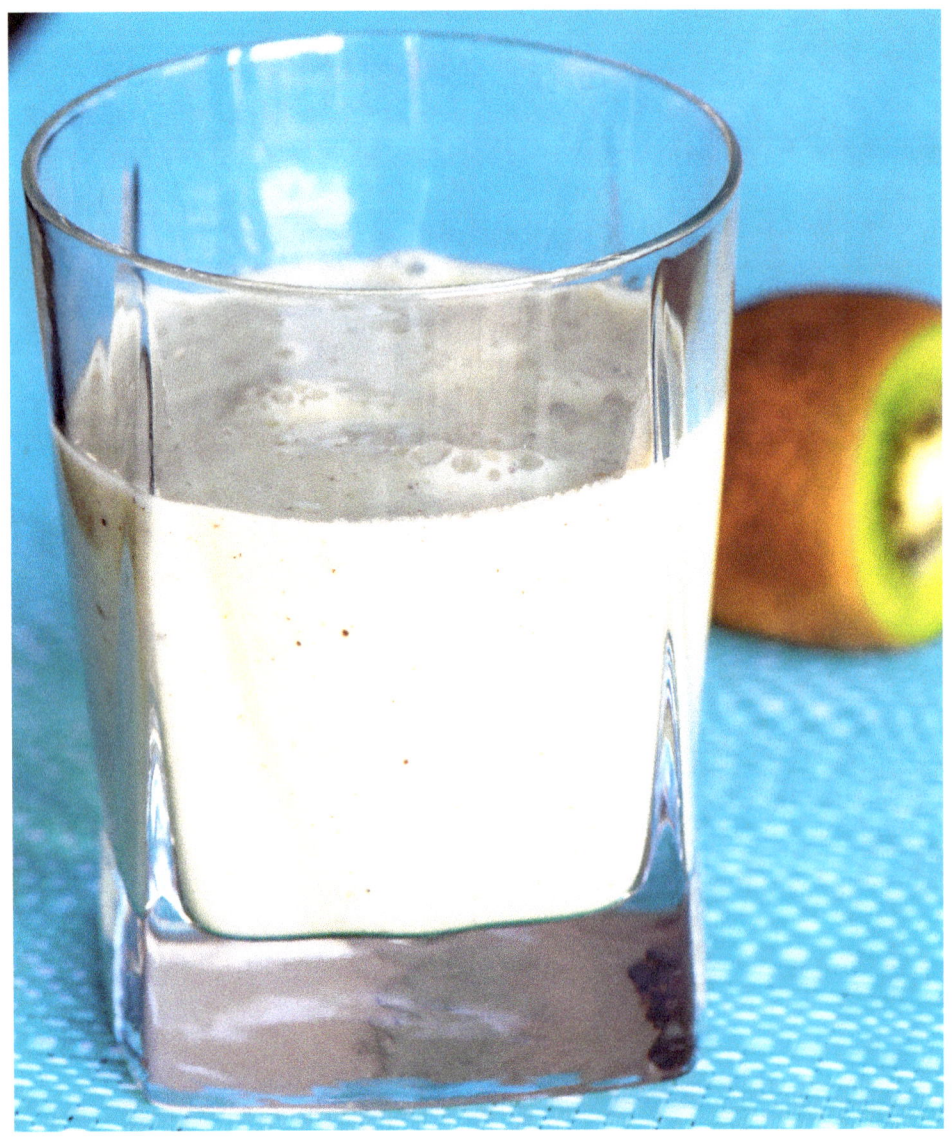

Prep time: 5 mins | Serves 1

A refreshing, slight tangy flavour from the Kiwifruit.
Kiwis are also full of nutrients like vitamin C, vitamin K,
vitamin E, folate, and potassium.

WHAT YOU'LL NEED:

1 kiwifruit

1 avocado

½ cup of natural yoghurt

½ cup almond milk

6-8 ice cubes

WHAT TO DO:

- Peel kiwifruit. Peel avocado and remove seed.

- Simply place all ingredients in a blender and blend until smooth.

Green Protein Smoothie

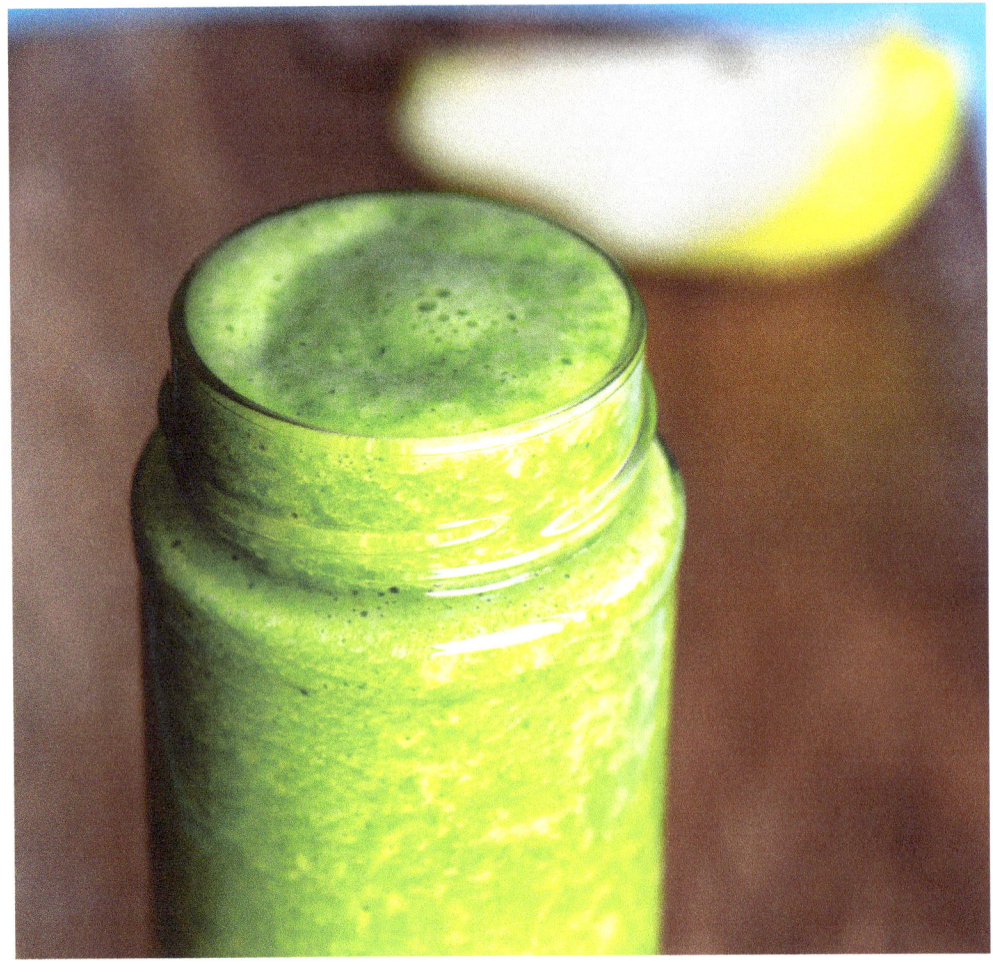

Prep time: 5 mins | Serves 1

For the green smoothie lover. A perfect way to pack your body full of all the nutrients found in greens.

WHAT YOU'LL NEED:

1 cup baby spinach

1 cup almond milk

1 pear

1 scoop of protein powder

¼ tsp. greens powder

WHAT TO DO:

- Remove core from pear.

- Simply place all ingredients in a blender and blend until smooth.

Greens powder is a way to boost the vitamins your body needs from green vegetables and grasses. It does have a bitter taste, so use sparingly until you get used to it.

Banana Honey Smoothie

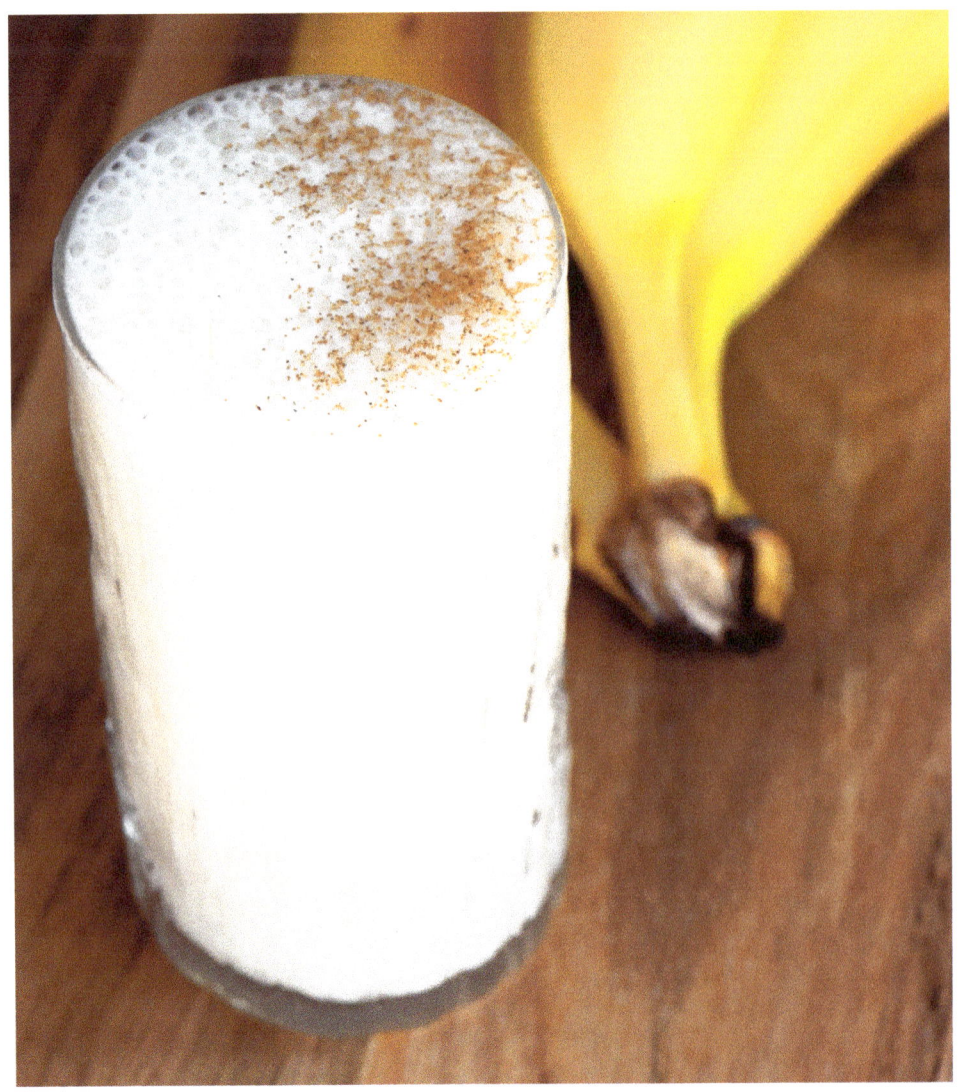

Prep time: 5 mins | Serves 1

A basic staple smoothie, and it will also be a hit with the kids. Start your day well.

WHAT YOU'LL NEED:

1 banana

1 cup milk

1 tbsp honey

Pinch of cinnamon

Pinch of nutmeg

½ scoop of protein powder

¼ cup of chia seed

WHAT TO DO:

- Peel banana.

- Simply place all ingredients in a blender and blend until smooth.

Chia seeds are known for their Omega 3 and fibre benefits. They are reasonably tasteless, and add a nice texture to any smoothie.

Raspberry Smoothie

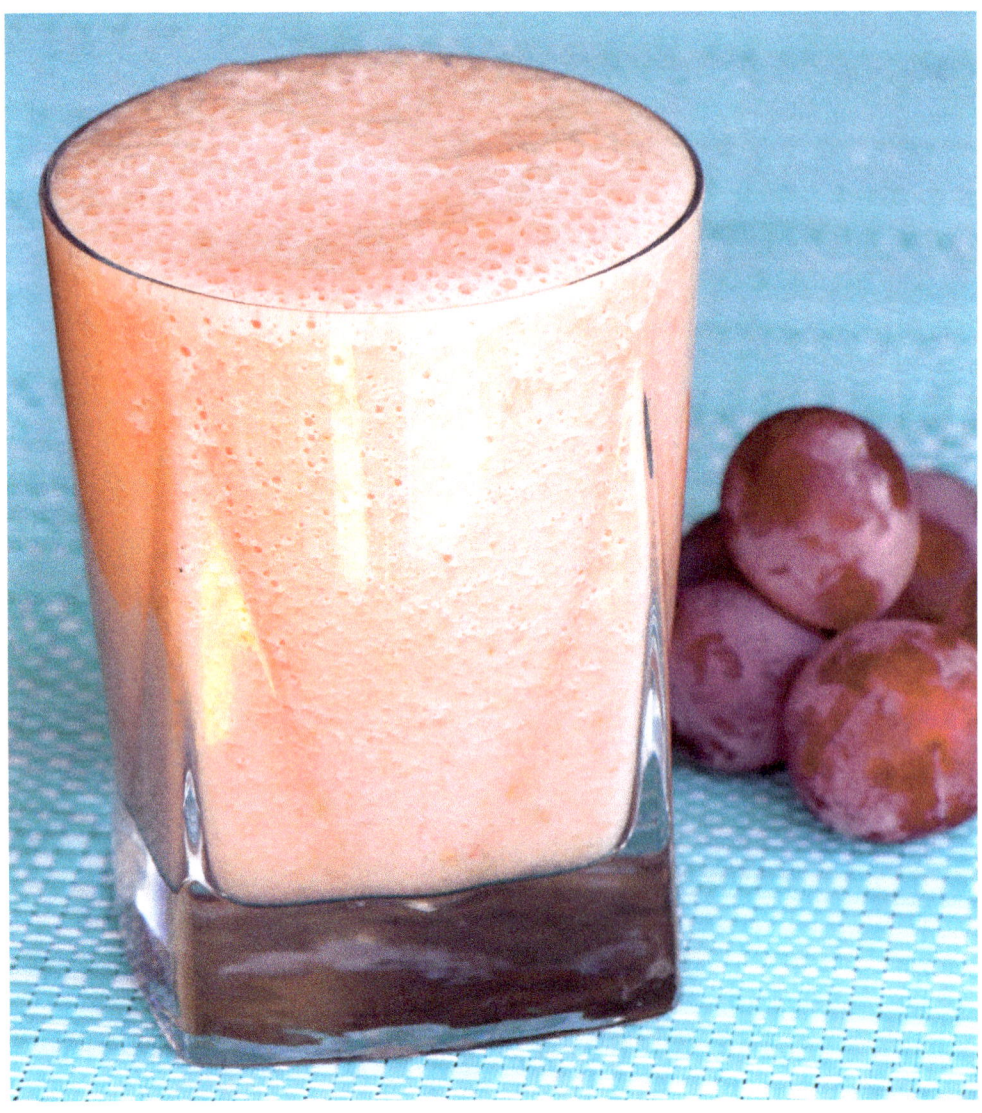

Prep time: 5 mins | Serves 1

A tasty refreshing smoothie, absolutely perfect for a snack.

WHAT YOU'LL NEED:

¼ cup raspberries

¼ of a banana

1 small carrot

1 cup of seedless grapes

½ scoop of protein powder

½ cup water

4-8 ice cubes

WHAT TO DO:

- Peel banana.

- Simply place all ingredients in a blender and blend until smooth.

Healthy Spinach Smoothie

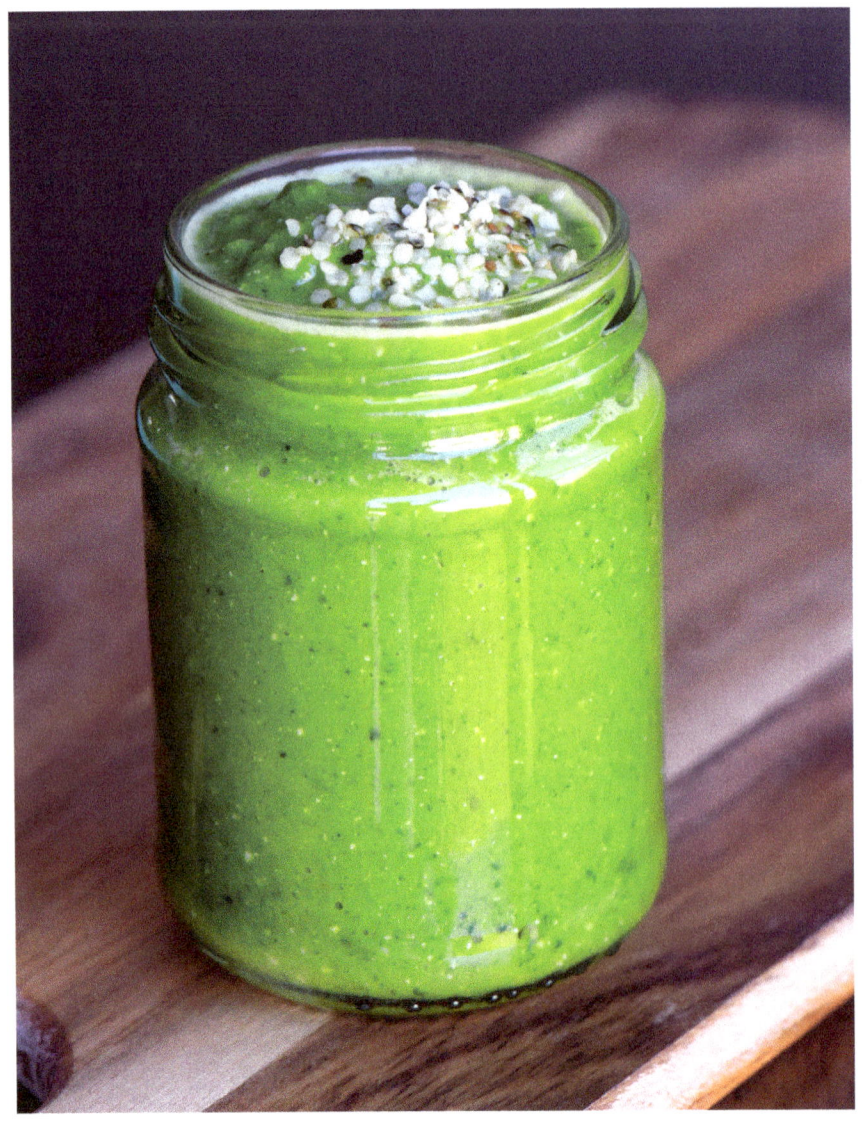

Prep time: 5 mins | Serves 1

You cant go wrong with green! Extremely easy way to raise your veggie intake, and reap the vitamin and mineral benefits.

WHAT YOU'LL NEED

1 cup baby spinach	1 apricot
½ an avocado	1 cup of water
1 cup of kale	¼ cup hemp seeds
½ a cucumber	6-8 ice cubes

WHAT TO DO:

- Peel and remove seed from avocado. Remove seed from apricot.

- Simply place all ingredients in a blender and blend until

Hemp seeds are high in protein and are full of essential fatty acids. They have a creamy nutty flavour and can be used in seed or powder form.

Just Peachy Smoothie

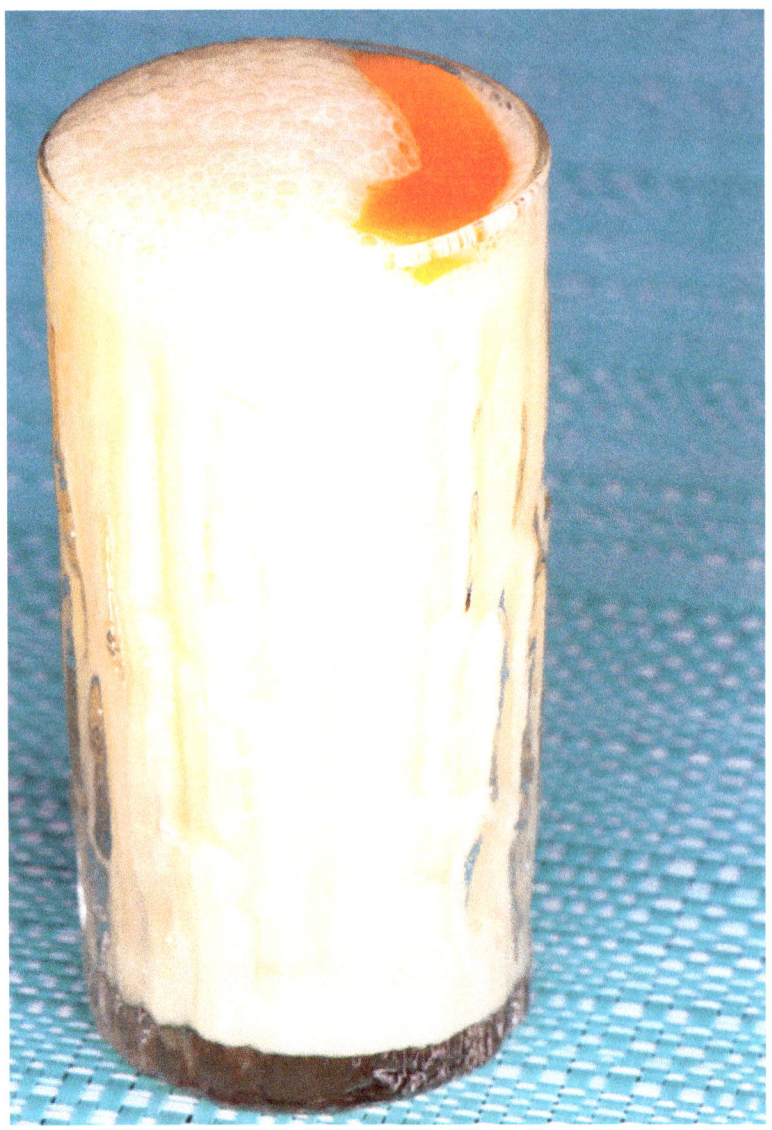

Prep time: 5 mins | Serves 1

The sweet flavour of the peaches will have you coming back for more. A great post workout drink.

WHAT YOU'LL NEED:

½ cup of peaches

½ cup natural yoghurt

½ tsp. powdered ginger

1 cup milk

6-8 ice cubes

WHAT TO DO:

• Peel and remove seed from peaches.

• Simply place all ingredients in a blender and blend until smooth.

If fresh peaches are not in season, substitute with canned ones.

Cacao Heaven Smoothie

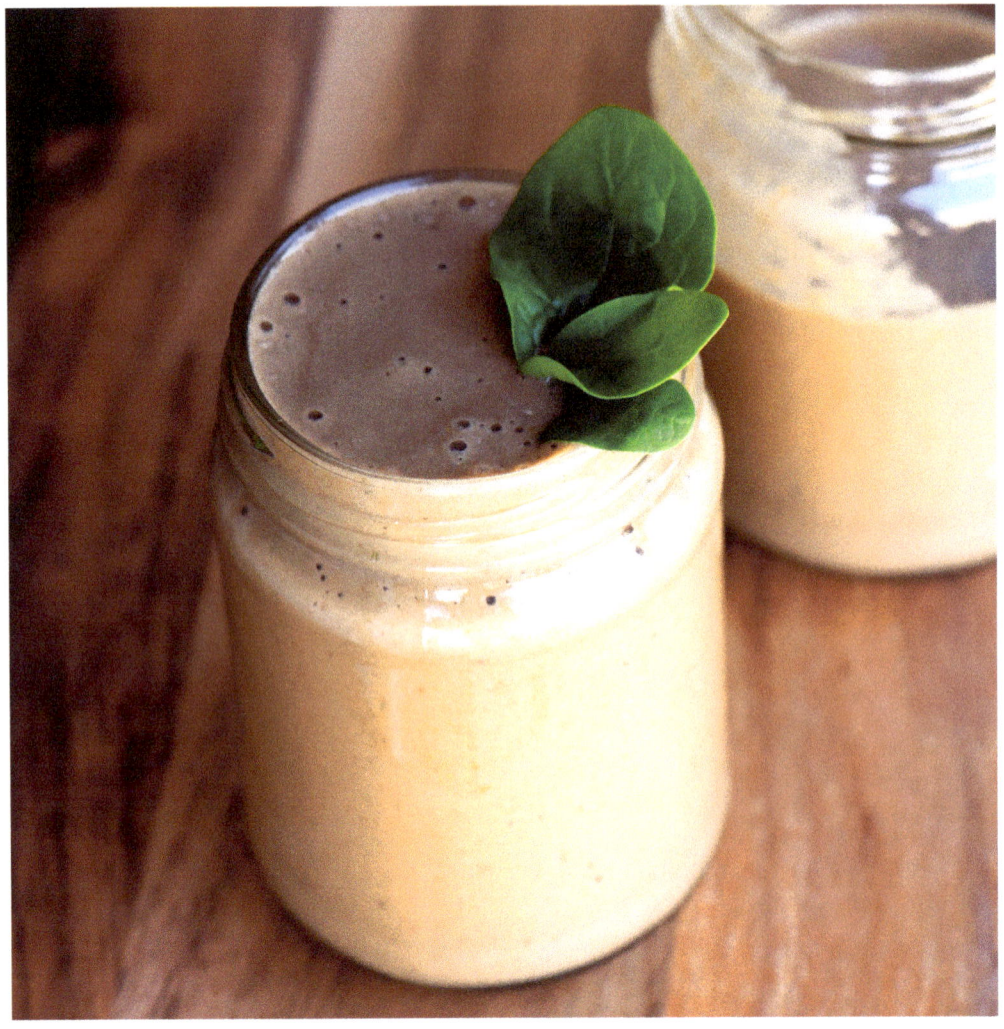

Prep time: 5 mins | Serves 1

Cacao is chocolate in its most natural form. A tasty chocolate flavoured smoothie thats so packed full of goodness its totally guilt free.

WHAT YOU'LL NEED:

2 tbsp. cacao powder

½ scoop protein powder

1 cup baby spinach

1 banana

1 cup almond milk

2 tbsp. hemp seeds

1 tsp. maca powder

6-8 ice cubes

WHAT TO DO:

- Peel banana.

- Simply place all ingredients in a blender and blend until smooth.

Raw cacao powder is known for its anti-inflammatory benefits. It has an earthy taste of dark chocolate. Cacao nibs can also be used for added texture.

Beetroot Cinnamon Smoothie

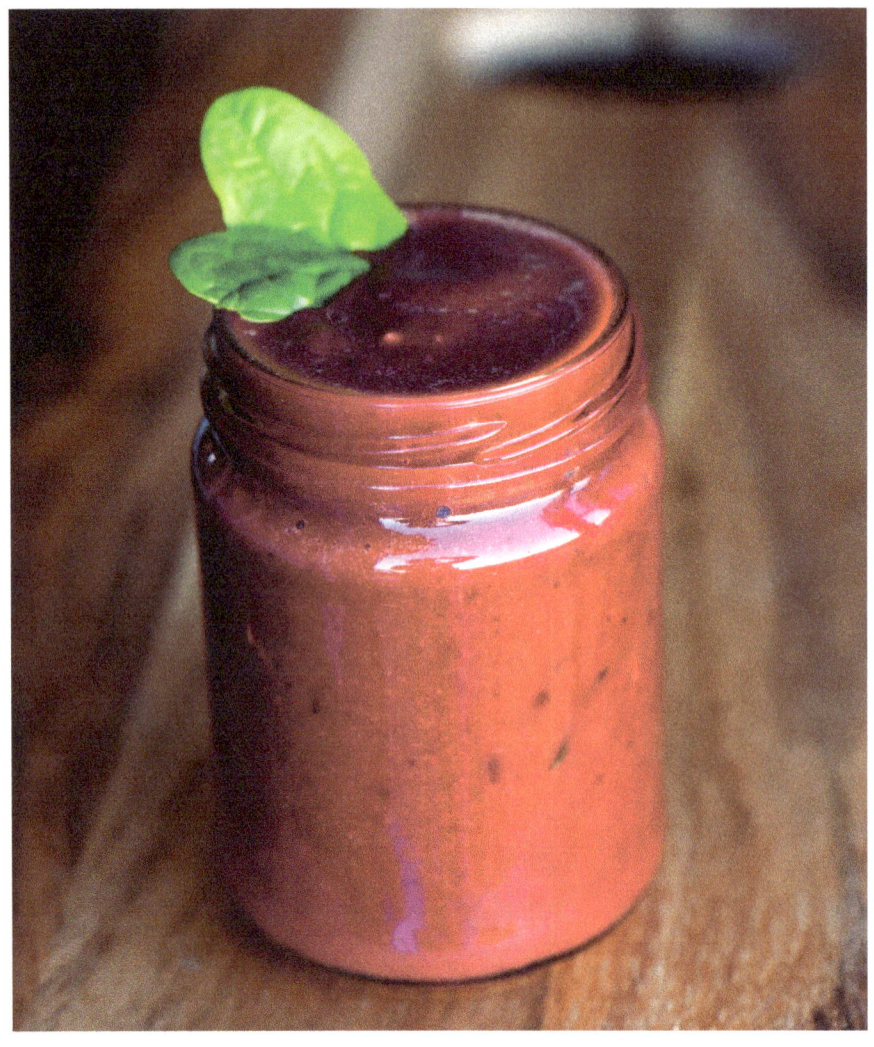

Prep time: 5 mins | Serves 1

This colourful delight is packed full of antioxidants, essential oils, vitamins and minerals. It's a whole glass of vitality all at once.

WHAT YOU'L NEED:

Handful of soaked almonds

1 avocado

1 banana

¼ cup of baby spinach

1 small raw beetroot

1 tsp. vanilla

1 tsp. honey

1 tsp. cinnamon

2 cups of water

WHAT TO DO:

- Peel avocado and remove seed. Peel and remove stem from the beetroot.

- Simply place all ingredients in a blender and blend until smooth.

Orange Mango Smoothie

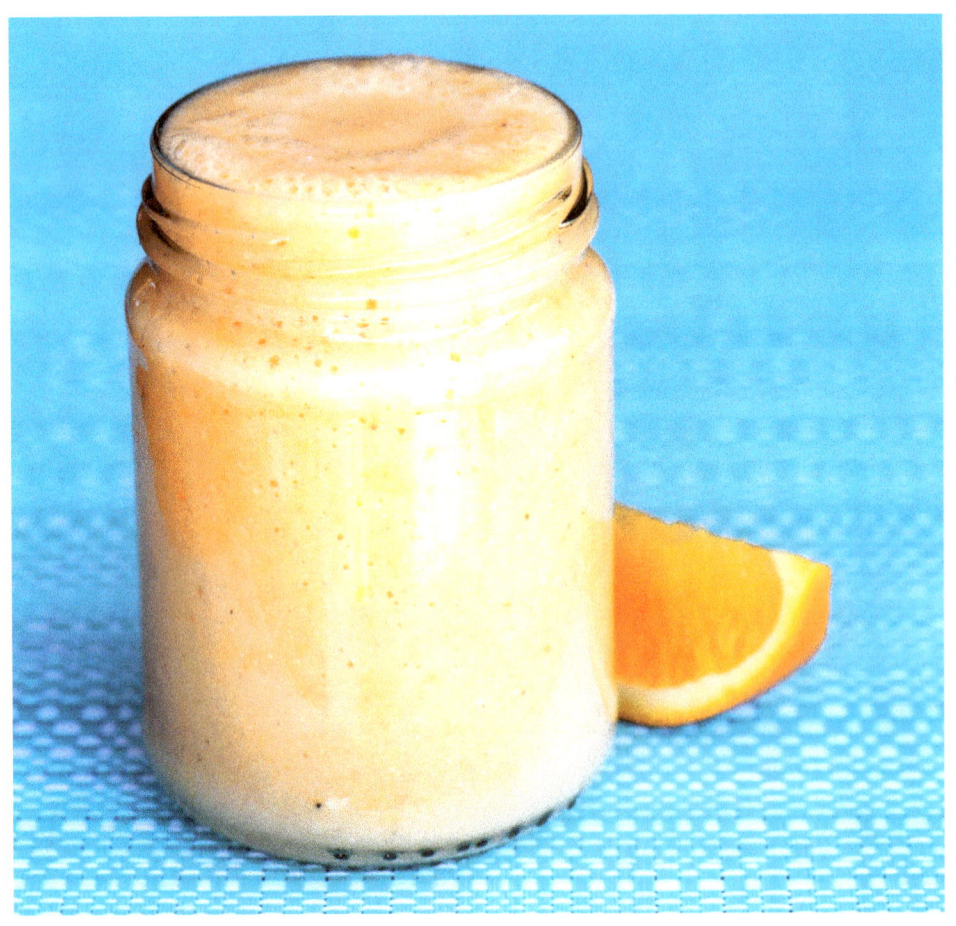

Prep time: 5 mins | Serves 1

A popular blend of flavours that is sweet and refreshing.
A perfect afternoon pick-me-up.

WHAT YOU'LL NEED:

1 orange	2 tbsp. hemp seeds
1 mango	½ a lemon
½ a carrot	1 cup almond milk
1 banana	6-8 ice cubes

WHAT TO DO:

- Peel and remove seeds from orange, lemon and mango. Peel banana.

- Simply place all ingredients in a blender and blend until smooth.

Carrot and Mango Smoothie

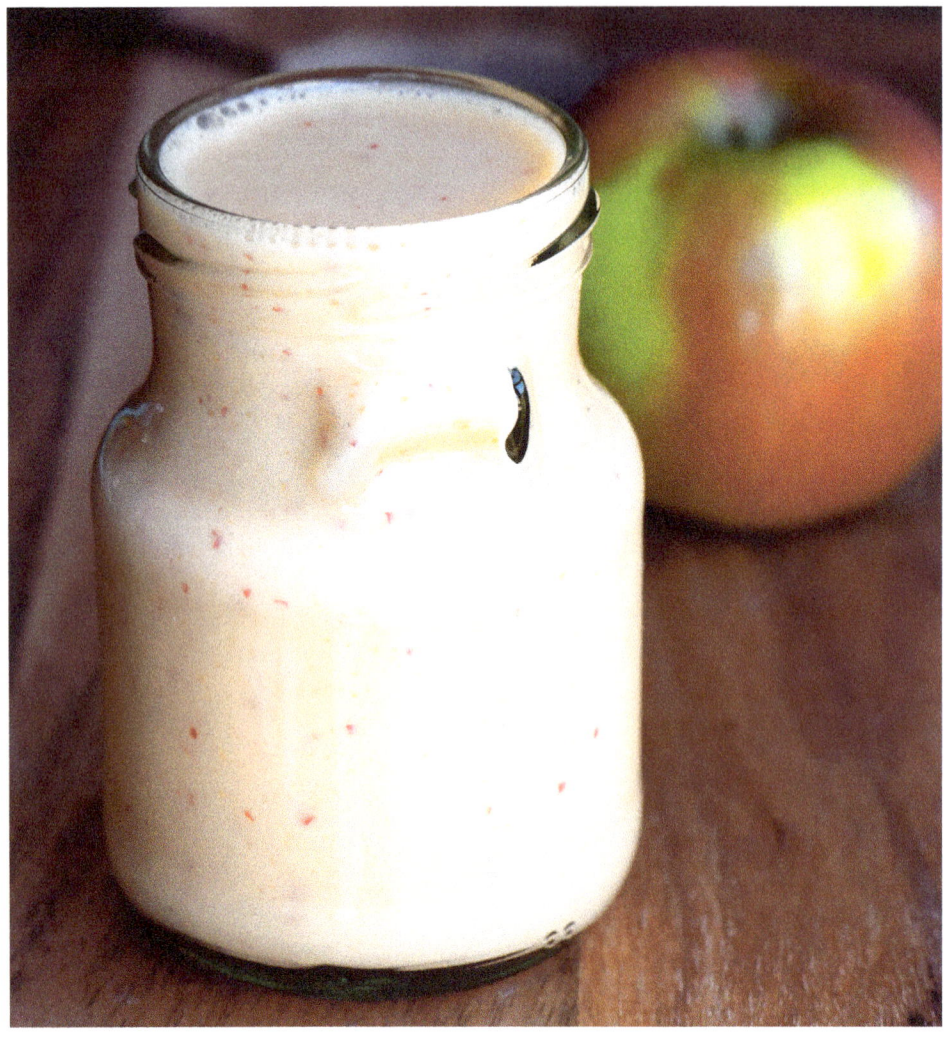

Prep time: 5 mins | Serves 1

Full of vitamin C, Vitamin A and Betacarotene.

WHAT YOU'LL NEED:

1 apple

1 small carrot

½ a mango

1cm piece of ginger

1 cup of natural yoghurt

WHAT TO DO:

- Remove core from apple. Peel and remove seed from mango.

- Simply place all ingredients in a blender and blend until smooth.

ALTERNATIVE:

- Juice the carrots, apples and ginger first.

- Blend the yoghurt and juice and refrigerate for 30 minutes.

- Stir and serve.

Blackberry Cheesecake Smoothie

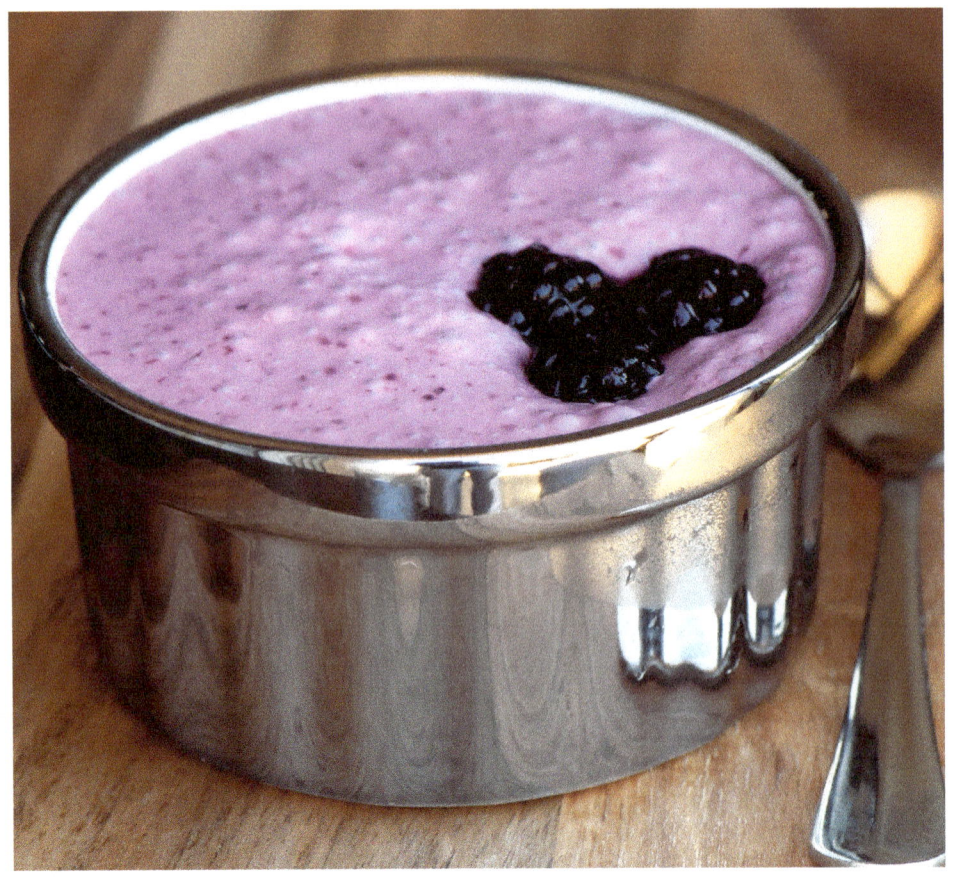

Prep time: 35 minutes | Serves 2

For the dessert lovers.
Perfect for a that occasional well deserved treat.

WHAT YOU'LL NEED:

1 cup frozen blackberries

1 cup thickened cream

1 cup cream cheese

2 cups of water

1 tsp. vanilla

WHAT TO DO:

- In a bowl, whip the cream until thickened. Stir the cream cheese until softened and then fold into the whipped cream.

- Blend the blackberries, water, and vanilla together. Gently stir the blended mix into the cream and cheese.

- Place into individual bowls and place in fridge for 30 minutes, then serve.

My Story

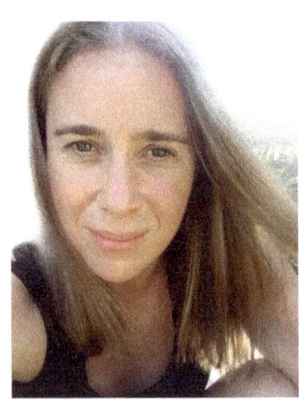

Hello, I am TJ, owner of Simplistic Nutrition and Health.

I am a mother of two amazing little people, with a passion for ultra marathon running and a strong sense of adventure.
I love nothing more than running through the mountains, and having a body that is healthy enough to allow me to do so.
I started in the fitness industry 15 years ago. I had the qualification, but I lacked the life experience.
Since those gym days, my outlook has totally changed. I now have a holistic approach to fitness, which involves finding the activity you love doing, and doing more of that. It doesn't matter whether that is organised sport, hiking, paddle boarding or getting outdoors and playing with the kids, its whatever you enjoy doing for you.
I take a non-diet approach to eating which means there are no restrictions and no counting calories. Eating in moderation and fuelling your body with balanced wholesome home cooked nutritious meals is all it takes.
Recharge your soul and the other elements of being fit and healthy will follow.

We get one chance at life, LIVE IT!

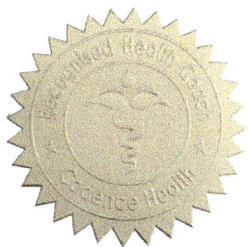 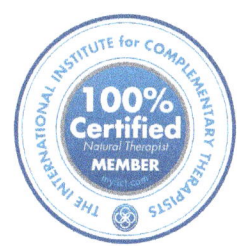

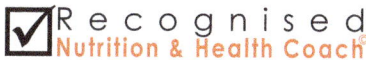

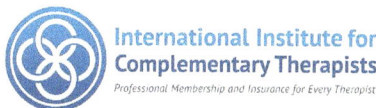

- Advanced Certificate in Nutrition and Health Coaching – *Cadence Health*
- Professional Certificate of Menu Planning – *Cadence Health*
- Certificate IV in Personal Training – *Australian Institute of Fitness*
- CHISMS Programs Certificate IV Special Populations Children and Adolescents – *Children's Hospital in Westmead, Institute of Sports Medicine*
- Certificate III in Group Exercise – *Australian Institute of Fitness*
- Certificate III in Gym Instruction – *Australian Institute of Fitness*

CPSIA information can be obtained
at www.ICGtesting.com
Printed in the USA
BVHW022043240619
551754BV00031B/1398/P